Managing Violence and Aggression

For Churchill Livingstone:

Senior commissioning editor: Alex Mathieson
Project manager: Ewan Halley
Project editor: Mairi McCubbin
Project controller: Derek Robertson
Design direction: Judith Wright

Managing Violence and Aggression

A manual for nurses and health care workers

Tom Mason RMN RNMH RGN BSc(Hons) PhD
Senior Lecturer in Forensic Psychiatric Nursing/Research,
Liverpool University, Liverpool, UK

Mark Chandley RMN BA(Hons)
Team Leader, Elms Ward,
Liverpool University, Liverpool, UK
Ashworth Hospital, Maghull, Merseyside, UK

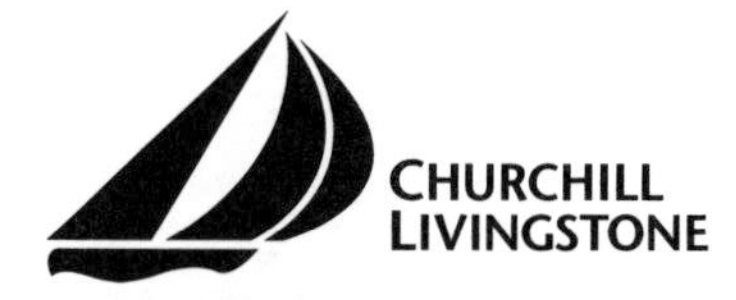

EDINBURGH LONDON NEW YORK PHILADELPHIA SYDNEY TORONTO 1999

Churchill Livingstone
An imprint of Elsevier Science Limited

First published 1999
Reprinted 2001, 2002

ISBN 0 443 05934 9

British Library Cataloguing in Publication Data
A catalogue record for this book is available from the British Library.

Library of Congress Cataloging in Publication Data
A catalog record for this book is available from the Library of Congress.

The publisher's policy is to use **paper manufactured from sustainable forests**

Printed in China by RDC Group Limited
B/03

Contents

Preface

The growing literature on violence and aggression would suggest a growing need to understand, prevent and control the harm, fear, pain and injury that they cause. The threat of violence is of concern to all members of society and more so to members of the health care professions whose task it is to care for those who are in need but who may also become violent. Those who attack others also tend to be hurt in the process and ultimately are brought into contact with health professionals either in casualty departments or psychiatric services. If the violent person has an accompanying disorder, such as a learning difficulty, mental disorder, personality disorder or drug addiction, then the aggression becomes part of the 'medical' problem and thus receives some form of intervention. Therefore, treatment of violence and aggression is of central concern.

The greatest consideration in dealing with violent persons is at the moment when actual assault takes place. At this juncture the main concerns are how to control the violence and how to avoid injuries. However, there are two other important moments, which are immediately preceding the violence and immediately following it. Here one encounters issues of how to avoid the violence, and how to prevent it occurring again. These reflect the focus of this book, in that its structure follows the lines of development of the occurrence of violence, as we look in turn at the phases prior to, during and following the crisis of combat.

We would also like to point out that throughout the book we refer to the violent person as 'he'. This is not out of a theoretical gender bias but merely for ease of writing and is justified on the basis that males are, generally, more violent than females.

Liverpool, 1998

Tom Mason
Mark Chandley

Acknowledgements

In a project that commands 'home time' the immediate thanks must go to our respective families. Both our wives, Helen and Jane, and our young children, Kelly, Lois and India Mason and Lewis and Ross Chandley, have given much support and tolerance in the long hours of writing.

Thereafter, a small group of friends have had a great influence. They include Dave Mercer, Les Jennings and all the staff who work on Elms Ward in Ashworth Hospital. Observing their practice is a book in itself.

A short statement also goes to others who have 'inadvertantly helped': thanks, but there is another way.

SECTION 1

General overview of violence and aggression

SECTION CONTENTS

1

Introduction

KEY POINTS

1. Some aggression is necessary for the survival of the human species.
2. It is a universal phenomenon existing in all cultures.
3. It is a question of cultural context as to what is considered to be acceptable levels of violence.
4. Fear is a natural response to violence and aggression.

INTRODUCTION

To understand the role of aggression in our society, and to reassure ourselves about the control and management of violent encounters, we need to appreciate that violence and aggression lie at the heart of humanity. The literature on violence and aggression has grown considerably over the years and is now considered to be comprehensive. This probably reveals two major elements relating to the role of violence and aggression in both the evolution of our species and the contemporary state of our global societies.

The first element is that violence and aggression appear to be either a close accompaniment to the emerging generic human, or a prerequisite for the rise of *Homo sapiens* as the dominant species of animal. This central role of violence and aggression in our development can be understood at a religious and mythological level; for instance there is the biblical account of Cain's killing of his brother Abel, very early in our creation, out of anger at falling from God's favour (Genesis 4: 8), as well as mythological accounts such as that of Bia, the god of violence, teaming up with Kratos, the god of force, both born of the Underworld, this battling of the divinities reflected in the life of humans (Graves 1986). It can also be understood at a more secular level with the evolutionary thesis offering us a more convincing argument that humans' faster developing brains, instinct towards herding, accumulation of strength through numbers, and our ingenious use of weapons gave us the developmental edge over other species. In any event, it would appear that as contemporary humans, we continue to be preoccupied with the same themes of violence and aggression, albeit in different forms, as were our ancestors.

The second element, referring to the vast literature on violence and aggression in contemporary society, may reflect the extent to which these remain universal problems requiring such intense effort to understand and overcome them. We seem to be torn apart with threats and dangers that permeate our lives, to the degree that we may actually be more surprised when we have not been attacked, than when we are.

There is a common understanding that not only is the human species inherently aggressive, but also that to survive in daily life, some proportion of aggression is necessary. Just as we are alarmed at the overt aggression of some people, so too, are we annoyed at those who refrain from 'standing up for themselves' or 'fighting back'. Those members of society who allegedly lack the required amount of forcefulness become the target of counselling and courses to correct their imbalance and learn to become more aggressive, although these courses are cloaked in the 'softer' expression of 'assertiveness training'. Therefore, there seems to be a middle ground of acceptable levels of aggression in which too little is almost as bad as too much. Similarly, in the case of violence, it is generally the accepted norm that some force may be necessary to protect either oneself or a third party, and again the question of degree is of central importance: turning the other cheek is one thing, raising one's arms to defend oneself is another, whilst striking someone in self-defence becomes an entirely different state of affairs.

Social encounters that incorporate the threat and tension of violence and aggression need navigating, as there are a series of social cues that are taken into account when assessing violent situations. Furthermore, such incidents are commonly followed by a process of psychosocial self-reflective critical appraisal, often undertaken subconsciously, by the individuals involved, which evaluates the conclusion to the encounter from the participant's viewpoint. Whether this need to evaluate the encounter is socially constructed or instinctively driven matters little. It is the evaluation of the perceived threat and the extent to which the response strategy used, employed an appropriate level of force that is important. We are all, no doubt, aware of encounters that have taken us by surprise and left us annoyed at having 'come off worst' in the verbal altercation. In rehearsing the scene in our minds, we tend to conclude 'I should have said this, or that, to them'. This individual evaluation is important in determining how we may respond in future situations.

Thus, we have a growing stock of knowledge of how we should respond to the violence and aggression that we meet in social encounters; this enables us to learn gradually how to deal with the different levels of threat to ourselves, and determines the extent of confidence in our responses, and also how satisfied our egos are in the social sphere. This leads to the question of what such encounters mean to us as social individuals. Before we move on to develop these themes, it is important to spend a few moments dealing with the semantics of some of the terms we will refer to in the remaining text.

DEFINING THE TERMS

Much of what is said in this book relies on a lay understanding of the different perspectives of all those involved in violence and aggression. As we will see later, these perspectives include those of the perpetrator, the target, the victim (who is not always the target), and others with a vested interest (family, friends, mental health professionals, police, etc.). Within this encounter, in which a number of people are drawn together, and which leads to, and involves violence and aggression, there is this lay understanding and a common language that provides the communication of this experience. This encounter is one that occurs in the 'everyday life world', and there are a number of 'arenas' that as members of our society we become familiar with, which include the school playground, the night club, the football terraces, and so on. Their familiarity enables us to analyse situations that are likely to become violent, assess confrontations that appear aggressive in nature, evaluate incidents that are threatening, and take evasive action to dangerous encounters. Generally, we also become adept at adopting strategies to manage these encounters, whether they lead to direct violence or not, and gain some advantage, even in the face of overt aggression. This advantage can be achieved by a reaffirmation of our own value system, or a portrayal of high moral order to a perceived audience. For example, this could be realised by responding to an aggressive situation with an equally aggressive manner legitimating this response as necessary, correct and proper. Similarly, one may ignore an aggressive encounter, which is portrayed as 'backing-down', but the moral ground is then claimed by devaluing the act of resorting to aggression. Understanding this interplay of social forces contributes towards our comprehension of violence and aggression in society.

The suggestion that violence and aggression can become medicalised or, more accurately, psychiatrised concepts makes them amenable to diagnosis, treatment and prognosis; it also implies that 'expertise' gained about them is located in professional domains rather than in social ones. However, medicalising violence and aggression strips them of their social understanding, location and management, and restricts the analysis to causative psychopathology, which in turn restricts the response strategies. This causes a tension arising from the fact that violence and aggression are, first and foremost, social elements in which we are all 'experts' or 'experienced'. Such a separation of lay and professional concepts is, we will argue, both inaccurate and unhelpful. It is our contention that lay and professional domains lie closer together rather than standing apart when we are dealing with the extreme social rawness of violence and aggression.

For the purpose of this text, we would therefore like to define some general terms in a conjoint social and professional language.

1. Violence – this can be defined as the harmful and unlawful use of force or strength; of or caused by physical assault. The violent person is commonly understood to be someone who attacks another. We use the term in this book to refer to someone engaged, or engaging, in assault on another person either with or without the use of weapons.
2. Aggression – for our purposes, this differs slightly from actual violence and refers more to a disposition to show hostility towards becoming violent, but clearly can also involve assault itself. Aggression is an extremely wide term with both negative and positive connotations. In this context we understand aggression to be an extreme negative tendency towards becoming assaultive.
3. Assertiveness – in general terms, assertiveness suggests a lesser degree of aggression by which someone puts himself forward either physically or verbally. However, in mental health circles, it is often defined in terms of confidence, non-aggressive communication, and not being related to power over others.
4. Volition – this refers to an act of free will preceding a physical movement. It is based on the idea that it is a voluntary mental selection of a particular action from a number of possible choices. We use the term to refer to an act that a certain person chooses to do of his own free will.
5. Free will – this general term suggests that behaviour is, to one degree or another, under the control of the will. That we act according to our wishes is a central theme of this philosophical concept.

These terms, then, have a meaning in both the lay context and the professional one; as members of society, we have all encountered violence and aggression in one form or another, and have learnt to assess and initiate avoidance of it wherever that is possible. As members of society, we are therefore all knowledgeable persons as far as manoeuvring in aggressive social encounters is concerned, and these skills are culturally specific – that is, they will differ from society to society and even between subgroups within a wider cultural entity. We intend to draw on these lay and cultural skills and incorporate them into our professional practice.

CULTURAL CONTEXTS

We are now aware that violence and aggression occur in all cultures, to one degree or another, which makes them universal phenomena. Hunter members of the animal kingdom rely to a large extent on violence and aggression for survival in the search for food and sustenance, and although a decreasing number of human populations continue as hunters in the truest sense, it may be that remnants of this hunting-based aggression remain in other human populations. Although this remnant is predominantly successfully suppressed and sublimated into expression through sports, hobbies and work, there are some people who erupt into violence through a loss of this control. In accounting for such eruptions we cannot rely solely on the theory of repressed hunting aggression becoming unleashed, as many factors converge to produce aggressive individuals; however, other contributing factors are themselves, often, culturally determined. For example, the USA is popularly perceived as a violent society whilst Austria is not.

What is interesting, however, is that cultural responses to those engaging in violence and aggression largely depend upon whether that particular society has medicalised these conditions or not. Where cultures assume that violence and aggression should fall within the confines of psychiatry then the disposal of the aggressor is, by and large, the same – that is, transportation, according to legislation, to a place of residency for the application of treatments. Similarly, for cultures that consider acts of violence and aggression to be antisocial criminal activity, the response is likely to be some form of retributive process. The commonality of the two approaches is that both are attempts to ensure that the person involved desists from further acts of violence and aggression. The fundamental principle in both types of system is to protect other members of that society from harm. This protection from harm lies at the psychosocial heart of all societies and governs their responses to acts of aggression in both psychiatrised and non-psychiatrised countries.

Let us look at the non-psychiatrised type of response. Westermeyer & Kroll (1978) reported on a study of violence, and the cultural responses to it, in a 'peasant society' in Laos in Indo-China. This country, at the time of the study, was without psychiatrists or psychiatric institutions. Persons in a Laotian village who became *baa* (crazy) and violent were subject to several responses depending upon the extent of *baa* and the degree of violence shown. This could be loosely translated as an assessment of the person's dangerousness by family members, and whether they were in need of some assistance. The Laotian people had two options available to them when they sought help, depending on their geographical location. If they were close enough to a police station, a police officer would be summoned and would assess (independent review) the *baa* person's requirements. The options ranged from restraints by holding, restraints by tying, restraints by chain, handcuffs and stocks, to incarceration in jail or a deep pit in the ground (seclusion). Holding the *baa* person may involve shifts of relatives and friends taking turns to hold the unfortunate person physically until he was calm (control and restraint, see p. 145); the restraint materials could include rope, bamboo pieces, wire, cloth, handcuffs or chains. There were also stocks made of logs of wood with spaces hewn out for placing over the legs of the seated *baa* person. If there was no police station in the vicinity, then the local monastery would be contacted, and a similar assessment function would be undertaken by the monks. The monasteries held the chains for the restraint and would loan them out to the family until the *baa* person was calm. Sometimes the monastery would take the violent villager into the monastery and keep him locked up until the violence dissipated (Westermeyer & Kroll 1978).

What is interesting in this non-psychiatrised account of the 'folk' management of violence is the appeal to the law (police station) and morality (monastery), which has similarities to our own psychiatric system involving the Mental Health Act (legislation) and the higher morality of treatment (psychiatry) over retribution. This suggests that just as violence is a universal phenomena, so too is the appeal to legal and moral frameworks. It appears that the human species is not only concerned with the extent of violence of other members, but also, that the control of such aggression should be correct and proper.

ROLE OF VIOLENCE AND AGGRESSION IN OUR SOCIETY

In our attempt at contributing towards an explanatory framework of the role of violence and aggression in our Westernised and psychiatrised society, we will focus on an examination of the macrosocial structures that give us a glimpse into the cultural soul in which they are rooted. Although an overview of theories of violence and aggression will be outlined in Chapter 2, in this introductory chapter we would like to concentrate on a narrow range of issues that contribute to our understanding of the role of violence.

First, there exists an 'economy of dangerousness' in which the production of fear is manipulated; this is then followed by the emergence of an 'industry of protectionism', which surrounds it. As members of society, we are all fearful of violence and aggression, and it is this fear that enables the image makers of dangerousness to ply their trade. For instance, much of the news on television is concerned with the fear of violence in its many guises, from the bomber who wreaks havoc on the unsuspecting public to the mugger who batters an elderly lady for a few pence, and from the mob rampaging through our streets to the lone stalker haunting an individual; the fear generated by these reports, which we all share, shakes the foundations of our society. The newspapers are forever watchful of our community, always on the lookout for our concerns, and diligent in manipulating a story that links into our fear, fuelling and fanning its flames. The industry of protection, too, is a growth economy. From the insurance companies insisting upon ever more security to the advertisements of burglar alarms insisting we are not safe, and from the spiralling crime rates to the security guards patrolling our shops, we become trapped into the images of an increasingly violent society.

In the popular imagination, much of the violence and aggression lurk hidden in the dark areas of the night or in geographical locations such as the seedier parts of our cities. However, the fact that each and everyone of us can stumble across it in the most apparently neutral arenas of social life heightens our tensions regarding violence and aggression. There is always a feeling that it is somewhere 'out there', implicit, hidden and invisible – at the supermarket checkout, the doctor's reception room, and the hospital waiting room. It is because so much violence and aggression lie hidden and beyond our authority that society appears to need to make them visible in order to control them. This is achieved by our production and voyeurism of them.

The number of violent films that have been produced and have been deemed successful in terms of box-office sales is vast. Their close-up shots and slow-motion scenes are testimonies to our need to see the intricacies of violence. Injuries that are made to look starkly real, and the emotions of pain and fear vividly expressed, evoke in us a sense of empathy, of being there, and yet also being here in our seats as voyeurs, safe from the encounter happening in front of our eyes. We have created the confrontation portrayed, albeit falsely, since it is merely actors and actresses playing out the scenes of violence and aggression, and on film we can relive it over and over again, perhaps in the hope that we can understand it, come to terms with it, control it and finally dominate it. This process is little different from the relationship that violence and aggression have with psychiatry; violence can be produced by psychiatry through its penetrating enquiry, compulsory detention, coercive interventions, paternalism and patriarchy.

RESPONDING TO VIOLENCE AND AGGRESSION

Responses to violence and aggression are numerous; some people become physically sick, whilst others develop emotional reactions. Although some find violence abhorrent, others may become psychologically excited, while still others become sexually aroused. However, the response that we wish to focus upon here is one grounded in fear as a reaction to the encroachment of violence and aggression, which is the most common reaction in the majority of people.

When confronted with situations of an aggressive nature we are all familiar with the 'fight' or 'flight' possibilities in response to the surge of adrenaline. However, taking the situation in its entirety we can see that there is a complex interplay of factors that contribute to our assessment of whether 'fight' or 'flight' should be undertaken. In meeting a violent encounter that creates fear in ourselves, there are a number of biological responses that occur in our bodies and over which we have little control. These are a result of the production of adrenaline, which has biophysiological reactions that are transmitted into our everyday experience of the dangerous situation. These responses and reactions can be tabulated accordingly (Box 1.1). This production of adrenaline constitutes a reserve mechanism that is available to us in times of acute stress. Adrenaline is produced in response to danger or anger and prepares the body for action in abnormal conditions. It should be stated here that its effects are natural and without them we could be more vulnerable, that is, slower to react. However, it should also be noted that they constitute a highly charged state of readiness that can cause problems of overreaction and behaviour that would be deemed to be out of character. We will return to this point later in the book but wish to emphasise here their *normality*.

Box 1.1 Responses to fear

Biophysiological responses to adrenaline	*Resultant everyday/lay experience*
Constriction of the arteries resulting in a rise in blood pressure	Blanching of the skin making you look as 'white as a ghost'
Increase in the rate of the heart	Heart thumping in the chest
Stimulation of the liver to convert glycogen to glucose	Excess energy produced
Relaxation of the involuntary muscles of the bronchi	More oxygen is taken in with deep breathing
Dilation of the pupils of the eyes	Can receive more sensory visual data but makes you have staring eyes
Reduction in the secretion of saliva	Dry mouth
Increase in the activity of the sweat glands	Sweaty palms, back, underarm, face
Contraction of the arrectores pilorum muscles in the skin	Goose-pimples
Contraction of the sphincters of the alimentary tract	A hollow feeling in the stomach

The physical/biological response to fear induced by a dangerous encounter cannot, however, be isolated from the social aspects of the situation in everyday violence. Not only do we assess social aspects of the encounter (which we return to later) but we also evaluate our response of 'fight' or 'flight' in relation to our social world. For example, in encountering a danger, and becoming fearful, we may wish to respond by exiting from the conflict but feel that we would be derided as cowardly if we did so. Or departing from the fearful situation might leave others in danger and we might find this intolerable. Therefore, we may override our drive towards 'flight' and stay to aid others. Similarly, we may feel that 'fight' is the dominant response but we hold it in check as others may be watching and there may be serious repercussions to this action should we undertake it. Our social analysis of the encounter may nullify the biological response, or it may not. It is the interplay of this dynamism that, we feel, constitutes the need for a book on options for the management of violence and aggression.

THE STRUCTURE OF THIS BOOK

In the next chapter we will give a brief overview of the historical aspects of violence and aggression but will not dwell on this aspect as it is adequately covered in other publications. The aim of Chapter 2 is to establish violence and aggression, and ultimately what we do about it, as a dynamic event whose typology and quality change over time. Violence and aggression, and our social response to them, is examined in relation to our past, our evolution up to contemporary times, and the value systems that underlie their management.

Our value systems formulate the legal and moral framework in which we operate. For instance, they are central to the choice of physical restraint as opposed to isolation techniques, and are culturally, and often organisationally, determined. Their relationship to the pragmatics of managing violence is appraised in Chapter 2. This provides a social legitimacy for the diverse approaches to controlling and managing violent people, from the elderly mentally infirm to the autistic child. As violence and aggression can be subculturally legitimated as normative behaviour, so too can the response to their control. However, this raises human and civil rights issues, which are examined in Chapter 2. The chapter concludes with an examination of the need to develop the themes of therapeutic interventions, control and management of the expansion of violence and aggression, and it looks at a number of relevant areas including settings from reception areas to accident and emergency rooms, and from community nursing to high-security psychiatric services.

In Chapter 3 we deal with the growth of institutions, organisations and professions that claim expertise in managing violence and aggression. The medicalisation (or psychologisation) of dangerous individuals is examined in detail as this is central to the theme of the book in marrying theory to the pragmatics of managing violent people. The industry surrounding the management of aggression is also dealt with in Chapter 3. Just as there are physical organisations in society for the control of violence, such as prisons, secure hospitals and specialist units, so also are there social institutions set up to control violence and aggression in the community, such as police, religions, security firms, community psychiatric nurses, social workers and so on. These, of course, require a social legitimation, which is briefly mentioned in Chapter 3; they are designed for the circumscription of dangerousness, which has provided the motivation for the abundance of published risk assessments. The latter are also briefly reviewed.

Finally in Chapter 3, the phases of violence and aggression are set out. These include phase one, in which a person is aware that he is in a situation that has the potential for violence occurring but is actually relatively normal at that time. In phase two, there is an awareness that the situation is deteriorating into a more likely physical encounter. Phase three includes the moment of attack and the person's response to this in terms of the options available.

Chapter 4 deals with the underexplored area of observation and surveillance of potentially violent situations. The importance of appropriate levels of observation will be explained and will include such concepts as close observations, intensive observations, special observations, one to one and so on. The skills required to engage in effective observations are discussed and the thorny issue of what exactly one is supposed to be observing will be explained. This will provide readers with a checklist of both lay and professional signs and symptoms to look for when in a situation in which they are responsible for managing potential violence. Surveillance, a more systematic and continued form of observation, will also be discussed in relation to the growth of technology. This area includes the appropriate use of alarm systems, electronic devices, closed-circuit television (CCTV), door alarms, and strategic mirrors. Finally, in Chapter 4, we will begin to explore some early de-escalatory techniques that can be adopted in phase one. Once one has observed 'something' amiss, there are strategies available to prevent the situation from worsening and these are discussed. The chapter also includes information on slow-down approaches, verbal de-escalation and speech patterning.

The subject of Chapter 5 is resources and staffing; this is an area of growing importance as services are increasingly preoccupied with the management of assets and with fiscal considerations. The balance between adequate resources and staff/patient safety is a finely tuned one with disastrous consequences when imbalance occurs. We explore this issue in three areas. First, we outline the environmental resources that may be required including the design of areas in which violent encounters may take place. This develops the theme begun in an earlier chapter dealing with the facilities that can be employed for the protection of staff and others in the locality. The notion of environmental manipulation is explained, and the importance of an awareness of surrounding factors contributing to the escalation of violence, is discussed. Second, staffing resources are examined in relation to the benefits of increasing or reducing quantities of staff, as both alternatives have a role to play, not only in the de-escalation of violence and aggression, but also in their control and management. We also debate other issues within staffing resources such as the level and experience of staff, the quality of interpersonal styles and the situations in which they are used. Third, space and time are outlined in terms of their implication as resources for the management of aggression; there has been a lack of development in this area but if correctly used, they can act as valuable resources to prevent serious injuries.

Chapter 6 develops the situation and discusses the interventive options that are available in phase two. In this phase, any number of interventive strategies aimed at preventing further aggression may be attempted. These include diversional activities such as physical outlets, social activities and distracting techniques. Behavioural-type interventions are discussed including behaviour modification, aversive treatments, differential reinforcement of other behaviour (DRO) scheduling, moral reasoning, etc. Specific interventions also include self-soothing skills, education, stress-reducing strategies, anxiety control and many others. Communication and verbal strategies are also addressed and include negotiation, positive social learning, tone of voice, verbal orientations and so on. Finally, it is important to ensure that the foregoing interventions, of which there are many more, are debated in relation to the practicalities of controlling and managing violence and aggression in the context in which they are set.

As the potentially violent situation worsens, and the likelihood of aggression becomes more imminent, then considerations need to be made as to the options available in this phase. Chapter 7 concentrates on the controlling measures that are accessible and how these should be managed. From the practical guidelines of policy formulation to the face-to-face confrontation, the issues discussed include verbal, contact and extended controls, short contacts and intensive observations. The chapter also develops the notion of raising confidence levels by providing the correct degree of control in the least restrictive circumstances. Other issues discussed in Chapter 7 include countertransference concerns, agreeable safety considerations, and the potential use of techniques for the removal of the aggressor. Included also, is an extensive coverage of management techniques of violence and aggression relating to crisis intervention, establishment of baseline behaviour, identification of attitudes, anticipation and making sense of aggressive behaviour. Finally, the predesign of preventive and reactive strategies and their importance in the control of violence and aggression are discussed.

Unfortunately, with the best will in the world, sometimes violence and aggression do occur, and in phase three it is important for control and management that knowledge and skill acquisition is achieved. In Chapter 8 we explore how the violent person can be isolated to prevent causing harm to others although he may destroy property. The various types of seclusionary practices are highlighted and practical suggestions made for emergency control. The issues involved in the practice of isolating patients are then discussed and the problems that it can raise are aired. An appropriate plan of action is offered to forestall problems and help with quick and effective control and management of the violent person. Such a 'plan of action' must be seen in context and be relevant to the individual organisation; however, there are central themes that emerge and overlap in particular situations. The advantages and disadvantages of different methods of seclusion for different client groups are outlined and an examination is made of alternative approaches.

Physical restraint is a very basic response to being attacked and is fundamental to defence. In Chapter 9, it is deemed not only elementary to survival but also part and parcel of our legitimated codes and laws. Shedding the niceties of moral outrage and the embellishments of language, we deal with the core value of such restraint in the crisis of combat and protection of oneself and others. Chapter 9 deals with the 'rules of engagement' that must be followed in order to shield oneself from both the limitations established in law and the duties verified by professional qualifications. We include a discussion of the practical ramifications of such theoretical techniques as Control and Restraint (C&R), which is the Home Office-approved training programme for the physical control and management of violent people in prisons. This programme has now been introduced into a number of secure health care settings as well as in a number of general psychiatric facilities. Since its inception in psychiatry in the mid 1980s, it has developed into a more subtle intervention for the management of violence. Other physical restraining techniques are also dealt with in practical terms; they include gentle holding, bearhugging and pindown. Finally, the use of certain equipment such as blankets, mattresses and quilts as an aid in the physical control of violent individuals is also raised.

Chapter 10 takes us further into the practical difficulties of control and management of violent people, especially those who continue to be aggressive when the other interventive strategies have been attempted and failed. Mechanical restraints are examined and discussed in relation to their practical applicability. Such restraints include seat belts, bed rails and sheets, as well as bandages, special chairs and illusory devices. Also discussed are the use of mechanical restraints including straitjackets, camisoles, wristlets and Posey belts, along with protection nets, waist and pelvic restraints, spit shields and two/three/four-point restraints. The ethical difficulties are discussed in relation to the practical applications of all techniques in this difficult phase. Finally, we discuss preventive aggression devices (PADs), ambulatory restraints and decompression. These are longer-term issues that receive a full and frank discussion.

The central concern in Chapter 11 is the chemical control of the violent and aggressive person. Although the therapeutic role of drugs is briefly discussed, this is not the main focus of the chapter as it is adequately covered in many excellent texts. We focus rather upon the use of medication in the emergency situation, shortly before, or at, the crisis of combat.

For example, we outline the use of pro re nata (PRN) medication prior to the situation deteriorating to an assault, and the effective use of this form of prescription in preventing violent outbursts. Rapid neuroleptization and intravenous medication are outlined at the point of a violent incident occurring, when the patient continues to fight, and when the situation needs to be brought under immediate control. The advantages and disadvantages of chemical control in the violent situation are discussed, as are the practical implications for staff attempting to control a struggling patient. In all these situations, there are consequences for all those involved as when things go according to plan little notice is taken; however, when things go wrong there could be serious litigation as a result.

Chapter 12 presents a number of specific situations that call for specialist knowledge and skill. These situations are rare but cause a good deal of concern if they do occur. It is therefore important to discuss the many factors that contribute towards these complex situations as many staff can note aspects of them that can be extracted as useful information to incorporate into their own practice areas. The circumstances discussed include the hostage situation, in which another's life is at stake, the barricade, in which certain groups are isolated but unobtainable, the protest, which could for example be a rooftop incident, faecal smearing, or hunger strike. The role of negotiation is discussed together with the need for a further increase in staff skills and knowledge of repertoires.

In Chapter 13 we discuss the types of injuries that are predominantly caused in the immediate control and management of violence. We also raise points of first aid and the function of support in the overall role of carers. This involves a discussion of long-term problems caused by injuries sustained at the workplace as a result of violence by another. The role of the environment in the control and management of violence and aggression is well researched; the notions of chronic and acute stress are also explored. The role of fear in people managing aggression, and the response to it, is central to our discussion of aggression management. The production of safe and healthy working environments is also debated and an examination undertaken of which surroundings are best for the management of aggression. Finally, in Chapter 13, burn-out is recognised as a response to stress at work, particularly when the management of aggression is a feature of the work role; this can have a detrimental effect on the person's entire life structure and is not merely restricted to his or her workplace. We discuss signs and symptoms of burnout, the response to it and the ways in which it could be prevented.

The final chapter includes a discussion of how we can improve our knowledge and understanding of the control and management of violence and aggression. If we are to improve our ability to intervene effectively at an early stage, and also hopefully avoid the explosion of the attack, then we need mechanisms by which we can learn. These mechanisms are highlighted and include such techniques as supervision, education and research. Chapter 14 a lso includes an examination of the postincident review in which members of the multidisciplinary team, possibly including the patient, meet to discuss the events leading to the incident and explore ways in which it could be prevented in the future. Other models are also outlined and there is a discussion of the factors contributing to the display of violence and the role of staff in its management; this approach develops any lessons to be derived from such incidents. Other strategies debated include reflective practitioner approaches, the conducting of seminars, and workgroups. A final conclusion embraces the gaps in our knowledge base and explores future directions for the effective control and management of violence and aggression.

OVERALL THEME OF THIS BOOK

As was stated at the outset, much has been written on the topic of violence and aggression. However, for those who face people who are aggressive and are becoming violent, it is the practical consequences that are foremost in their minds. Health care employees require practical knowledge and skills to understand, avoid, reduce and manage the growing problem of violence and aggression in many walks of life. The theoretical perspectives on violence and aggression are important as they may inform us at the time of an incident occurring; for example, the theory of toxic confusional states may well have implications for how we deal with aggressive patients in this state. However, at the actual time of combat, it is the practical skills and knowledge that take precedence over the niceties of theory. This book is concerned with the practicalities of managing violence and aggression with a focus on avoidance, destimulation and the options available in the varying stages and types of aggressive situations.

The book is structured so as to take the issue of violence from a distance and analyse it as it becomes ever closer, through each successive chapter, until the aggression explodes into actual attack. This build-up, through the chapters, to the aggressive outburst should provide a sense of tension for the reader, which is similar to the tension facing those in the clinical arena. Thus, the theme of the book is to focus on the options available to those facing violent and aggressive individuals from a practical point of view. It is for this reason that Section 2, of the book, containing eight chapters, is concerned with the pragmatics of confrontation and combat. However, to increase our options, in terms of knowledge, understanding and providing a legitimation, we need also the information contained in Sections 1 and 3. Section 1 is concerned with violence and aggression *before* they occur whilst Section 3 deals with learning experiences *after* the event. Both Sections 1 and 3 should be read to support the central element dealing with the options.

2

The dynamic of violence and aggression

KEY POINTS

1. The theories and antecedents of violence and aggression are extensive.
2. Violence and aggression can be displayed by children, adolescents, adults and the elderly.
3. There is a wide range of clinical conditions that can manifest aggression.
4. The values of the society in which violence occurs governs our response to it.
5. Our professional responsibilities influence the values underpinning our management of violence.
6. It is the management of the encounter that creates danger and fear.

INTRODUCTION

In the previous chapter, we began to set out the role of violence and aggression in human societies and introduced some cultural contexts from both psychiatrised and non-psychiatrised communities. We understood violence and aggression to be central to many species' survival and although, in humans, this may no longer be the case in real terms, we could see many forms of sublimated aggression in sports, business and entertainment. We also noted that a certain degree of aggression was the accepted norm in many societies, with too much assertiveness being seen as just as problematic as too little. Furthermore, we drew attention to the fact that, just as a certain amount of aggression was considered 'normal' in our society, it was equally appropriate for others to respond to it in defence. However, this response also had to be within the parameters of what is considered to be 'normal'. In evolutionary terms, many species have developed hormonal responses to acute danger, and in humans, this includes the production of adrenaline to prepare the body for 'fight or flight'. The latter are two options that are available to most species of animal, including humans, when facing circumstances in which danger is perceived. This situational perception is what we know as fear; therefore, fear must be understood as a natural response to the perceived danger of violence and aggression.

In this chapter we wish to focus on the situational dynamic of violence and aggression. By this, we mean those factors that contribute towards our perception of a potential or actual violent encounter. When we perceive such an encounter, we undertake a series of evaluations that include the extent of danger, the amount of fear felt, and the options available in terms of response. In this dynamic, there are many such factors that are brought to bear on our evaluation. For example, we may well have a particular theory as to why a person or situation is deemed to us to be dangerous, which may, or may not, concur with another person's assessment of the same situation. What is important, however, is that one person's perception of danger is real to them, irrespective of any number of contrary evaluations by others, although the person may well be relieved, to some degree, by the reassurance of alternative views. This chapter, then, will deal with these situational aspects.

Firstly, we will give a brief overview of the theories of violence and aggression. However, it should be noted here that there is a plethora of work in this area with many excellent publications; therefore, we will merely offer a brief sketch and refer the interested reader to specific references. Secondly, we will broaden our understanding of the dynamic mentioned above by exploring both the fear and anxiety felt in this situation and the cultural responses available to us. This discussion then revolves around the socialised roles, values and norms from our respective cultures, which forms the third strand to the chapter. Fourthly, we will then set this into our understanding of contemporary violence and aggression in our society and briefly map out some underpinning assumptions to these aspects. Finally, we will locate the foregoing into health care settings, which adds another dimension in terms of the options available to us in violent encounters.

THEORIES OF AGGRESSION AND VIOLENCE

Blackburn (1993) identified differences between theories of aggression and antecedents of aggression. These, he argued, rested on different sets of assumptions, so that our understanding of the nature of aggression varied depending upon the emphasis placed on whether: (a) the components of aggression were either learned or unlearned, (b) the determinants were internal or external and (c) the processes were affective or cognitive. He stated that: 'they therefore differ in how they address the critical questions of how aggressive tendencies are acquired, maintained, and regulated, and how acts of aggression are "triggered" or provoked' (Blackburn 1993, p. 216).

The theories of aggression can be summarised according to several perspectives (Table 2.1).

Evolutionary perspectives

Firstly, there are the evolutionary perspectives, which suggest a universal instinct of aggression (Lorenz 1966) and in which comparisons to ethological studies have suggested that apparently innate energy sources govern human responses to external stimuli. However, such 'energy sources' have yet to be located. Evolutionary neurological scientists have also theorised on the sources and mechanics of human aggression in terms

Table 2.1 Theories of aggression

Perspective	Study	Theory
Evolutionary	Lorenz 1966	Instinct
	Moyer 1981	Chemical and electrical brain discharges
	Monroe 1978	Limbic damage
	Schalling et al 1987	Inhibition of MAO
	Widom & Ames 1988	PMT and diminished responsibility
	Virkunnen 1988	Hypoglycaemia
	Lidberg et al 1976	Adrenaline/noradrenaline
	Wilson 1978	Sociobiological explanations
	Moyer 1981	Ethological studies
Psychoanalytic	Freud 1920	Psychic conflict
	Kutash 1978	Ego weakness and acting out
Behavioural	Zillman 1979	Instrumental/angry aggression
	Dollard et al 1939	Frustration–aggression hypothesis
Social cognitive	Bandura 1982	Reinforcing contingencies
	Novaco 1978	Anger as stressor
	Averill 1982	Mental/physical/social dysfunction
Sociological	Wolfgang & Feracutti 1967	Subculture of violence
	Merton 1939	Anomie
	Pearson 1983	Football hooligans
	Tedeschi 1983	Exchange theory/coercive power

of neurochemical transmitters, electrical brain stimulation and organic lesions. These theories appear to suggest that organised neural circuits are triggered by chemical and/or electrical components, and produce specific attack behaviour (Moyer 1981). This idea is supported by the dyscontrol theory in which aggression follows loss of control as a result of limbic damage (Monroe 1978), testosterone inhibition of the enzyme monoamine oxidase (MAO) (Schalling et al 1987), premenstrual tension (PMT) and diminished responsibility (Widom & Ames 1988), hypoglycaemia (Virkunnen 1988), or altered adrenaline and noradrenaline levels (Lidberg et al 1976). Other evolutionary theorists include sociobiologists who believe that social behaviour is an amalgam of emotional responses; these include self-reflection and overt behaviours under genetic control that enhance the probability of the survival of the species at both a community and individual level (Wilson 1978). Also falling within the evolutionary perspective are ethological accounts which compare animal aggression and human aggression (Moyer 1981). However, these are often criticised on the grounds that there is little relationship between human behaviour and animal aggression (Blackburn 1993).

Psychoanalytical perspectives

Secondly, there are psychoanalytical perspectives; these comprise analyses of theoretical models of the human psyche, rather than investigations of organic and chemical structures of the body. The founder of psychoanalysis, Sigmund Freud, saw aggression as a response to pain and frustration. He developed the idea that the elements of the human mind were in conflict with each other, but that mental mechanisms in healthy individuals allowed for a resolution of these tensions. Aggression, he stated, was an instinctual aspect of the human in that, Thanatos, the death instinct, which was a tendency to destroy oneself, could be diverted by Eros, the human counter-mechanism for self-preservation (Freud 1920). Many later psychoanalysts have shed, to one degree or another, certain aspects of Freud's theory, but tended to maintain the notion of an aggressive instinct. The major thrust of psychoanalytical theories of aggression revolves around the idea that many behaviours are said to be a result of unresolved conflict in the mind, or an imbalance of control by the superego. The problem with psychoanalytical theories is that they can encompass almost every human aspect within their framework without any empirical testing.

Behavioural perspectives

Thirdly, there are behavioural perspectives. These are based on learning theories in which human aggression is acquired and maintained through reinforcements and punishments in social life. Within this overall theoretical framework, two types of aggression have been identified: *instrumental aggression*, which is positively reinforced by the acquisition of something, say money or status, and *angry aggression*, which is assumed to be negatively reinforced by the alleviation of something, say frustration or aversive stimuli (Zillman 1979). Focusing upon the antecedents of aggression, Dollard et al (1939) developed the *frustration-aggression hypothesis* according to which, the thwarting of objectives is the antecedent of aggression, which is directed at the source of interruption. However, Buss (1961) argued that frustration may lead not to aggression, but to some other behaviour, and also that insults, threats to self-esteem, attack by others and pain, may all provoke aggression. Aggression in such learning theories is considered to have a close relationship with events and people in the environment; therefore these theories involve associations with the human mind and its constructs (i.e. frustration). This association leads us to the theories of cognitive mediation.

Social cognitive perspectives

The fourth type, social cognitive perspectives of aggression, considers how people think and the way in which their intrapsychic structures lay the preparation for evaluation of, and response to external reality. In Bandura's (1982) cognitive theory of aggression, there is a complex relationship between reinforcing contingencies of behaviour, which is obtained from observations of expected outcomes from social interaction. The consequences of this behaviour for the self are that there is an adjustment of one's standards through a system of rewards and punishments. Other social cognitive theorists have focused more specifically on anger as a stress reaction that causes mental, physical and social dysfunction (Averill 1982, Novaco 1978). However, the problem with this idea is that the source of anger itself may well be determined cognitively by processes of appraisal according to models of social behaviour (Lazarus 1991). In the assessment and appraisal of events in the natural social world, and one's own behaviour in relation to it, we are well aware of the extent of misjudgements and misattributions in the generation of emotional reactions.

Sociological perspectives

Finally, there is the sociological perspective. Sociologists, social psychologists and anthropologists have argued that violence and aggression can be understood only in relation to the social context in which it is set. There are many variations in social structures that influence aggression and space only allows here for a brief mention of a few. Wolfgang & Ferracutti (1967) have suggested that a *subculture of violence* based on a masculine gender identity was responsible for aggression in society. They argued that a 'macho' image comprising the values of excitement, status, honour and toughness provided the basis for the exercise of aggression. Merton (1939) had earlier argued that certain social structures: 'exert a definite pressure upon certain persons in the society to engage in nonconformist rather than conformist conduct' (p. 672). His theory of *anomie* stated that there existed an imbalance between individual goal-directed aspirations and the social structures that regulated and controlled modes of achieving these goals; the tension or conflict between these states could produce aberrant behaviour, which could include violence and aggression. Becker's (1961) paper on the anthropological notes of the concept of aggression suggested that it could be viewed as an inept attempt at self-affirmation of a fragmented ego, as well as a learnt cultural method of gaining self-value and socially recognised power. Pearson (1983) studied the violent behaviour of British football hooligans and showed how elaborate ritual strategies of taunting and gesturing with strict rule formations within groups actually minimised physical attacks between rival supporters. He argued that this highly ritualised aggressive 'strutting' served to satisfy and contain aggression. Finally, Tedeschi (1983) argued that societies had reciprocal relations between the harm done to a victim and the retaliation expected in return. Through *exchange theory,* he argued that *coercive power* is used by those individuals who felt a need to maintain status, self-image and authority, in the face of the costs–benefits of addressing the inequitable social forces that maintained class division. As stated previously, in these types of theory the violence and aggression are seen in relation to the social context and it is assumed that these are normal within the culture that they are set in.

Other issues

In any comprehensive theoretical text on violence and aggression, one would expect to find some reference to particular issues such as violence and gender, and violence and race. However, as we intend to give only a brief theoretical overview of violence and aggression, and instead focus on the more practical issues, we will restrict ourselves to only a few comments on gender. The importance of the latter is not diminished by this; in fact, by highlighting them in our overview, we locate them as central to a contemporary understanding of violence in our society.

Gender and violence can be reviewed in a number of ways: males and females as perpetrators of violence, males and females as targets, sexual violence and domestic violence. However, the data on these areas are problematic as there are large areas of non-reporting and considerable confusion in the relationships between perpetrators and victims. For example, more males are killed than females per million population, except in the age bracket of 1–5 years, where they are equal (Levi 1994). However, killings by spouses or co-habitees puts females at greater risk in the ratio of 4 : 1

(Levi 1994). Thus, we see the complexities of relationship involvement. Furthermore, in turning our attention to sexual violence we see a growing complexity between rape of a stranger, rape within marriage, coerced sex, child sexual abuse, unwanted physical approaches, date rape, indecent assault, sexual harassment, etc. Suffice to say that this is, rightly, an area of intense research.

In this brief overview of the theories of aggression, it should be emphasised that there are many more available to the interested reader (for an excellent source see Blackburn 1993). Now we may begin to unravel some elements of the antecedents of aggression and violence.

ANTECEDENTS OF AGGRESSION AND VIOLENCE

Antecedents of aggression differ conceptually from theories of aggression in that the former refer, to some degree, to a causal relationship between the *tendency* towards aggression, and the *act* of aggression. If one has a tendency, or disposition, towards being aggressive then the antecedents are more likely to be distal – that is, causative factors occurring some considerable time before the event (e.g. environmental upbringing). However, antecedents of an act of aggression are more likely to be proximal – that is, life events or situational factors occurring directly before the aggressive act (Blackburn 1993). These types of antecedents are summarised as in Table 2.2.

Distal factors

If a person has a tendency towards aggression, then it can be said that they are likely to have developed this trait over a long period of time, probably from childhood. Although some longitudinal studies have shown this correlation (e.g. Feshbach & Price 1984), it should be noted that there is a high incidences of false positives (i.e. aggressive children who do not go on to become aggressive adults). It is now well established that early childhood experiences contribute to shaping the personality and, in longitudinal studies of aggression, early life events are said to be crucial in establishing this disposition. For example, some theorists, such as Buss (1961), have argued that childhood tendencies towards impulsivity, hyperactivity, overemotionality and independence, are antecedents to aggressiveness. If these signs are shown by children, they tend to increase the contact time with adults and siblings, and receive an excess of negative reactions in response to them. However, others have argued that parental deviance, marital conflict, indifference from parents, reduced supervision by parents, and parents who are harsh, punitive and erratic, are contributing factors (Cortes & Gatti 1972, Kolvin et al 1988, West 1982). It should be noted here that these terms suffer from a lack of definitional clarity, and also that family dynamics, as well as school experiences,

Table 2.2 Antecedents of aggression

Perspective	Study	Theory
Distal	Feshbach & Price 1984	Developed trait theory
	Buss 1961	Childhood impulsivity, hyperactivity, overemotionality and independence
	Cortes & Gatti 1972; West 1982; Kolvin et al 1988	Parenting factors/marital conflict
	Carney 1978	Lack of ability to trust
	Selby 1984	Anger
	Blackburn & Lee-Evans 1985	Self-esteem
	Kirchner, Kennedy & Draguns 1979	Social skills
	Huesmann, Eron & Yarmel 1987	Intellectual differences
	Toch 1969	Exercise of power
	Blackburn 1968, 1971; Megargee 1966	Over/undercontrolled personality types
Proximal	Lieber & Shervin 1972	Phases of the moon
	Mueller 1983	Environmental noise
	Anderson 1989	Climatic factors
	Rotton & Frey 1985	Ozone levels
	O'Neil et al 1979	Proxemic behaviour
	Mayhew, Elliott & Dowds 1989	Alcohol
	Pernanen 1991	Narrowing of perceptual field
	Buickhuisen, Van Der Plas-Korenhoff & Bontekoe 1988	Personality factors and alcohol
	Zimbardo 1970	Anonymity
	Wolfgang 1957	Victim precipitation
	Felson & Steadman 1983	Retaliation
	Berkowitz 1986	Face saving

are so wide and varied that it is difficult to pinpoint precise events that establish such aggressive traits.

Another approach is to attempt to understand aggressiveness in relation to the individual differences in the personal attributes of violent persons. This perspective is dependent upon identifying factors such as what such people consider to be aversive, or what makes them angry, frustrated and so on, and what coping mechanisms they have available to them in these situations. This view assumes that aggressive individuals have a certain lack of internal control. More specifically, Carney (1978) posited the view that: (a) aggressive individuals lacked the ability to trust, which was due to their poor role-playing skills; (b) they were unable to feel, which was evidenced in their acting-out behaviour; (c) they were unable to fantasise as seen in their impulsive behaviour; and (d) they were lacking in both empathy and learning skills, which was manifested in their inability to learn from experience. Other researchers have concentrated on the presence of anger as a trait (Selby 1984), differences in self-esteem (Blackburn & Lee-Evans 1985) and the level of social skills (Kirchner, Kennedy & Draguns 1979). There are also studies suggesting that intellectual differences may account for aggressive tendencies (Huesmann, Eron & Yarmel 1987), the argument here being that a person's intellectual development, or lack of it, may contribute towards social cognitive development, which is concerned with how children process information from their world.

Some considerable work has been undertaken on personality types and aggression. Toch (1969) proposed that violent persons fundamentally saw human relations as revolving around the exercise of power. From this he suggested that there were two broad interpersonal aggressive styles. One was based on personal feelings of vulnerability, self-preservation and defensiveness, whilst the second was manipulative, bullying and self-indulgent. Other workers on personality disorders have used the notions of over- and undercontrolled types (Blackburn 1968, 1971, Megargee 1966). The main thrust of such arguments is that overcontrolled aggressive individuals: 'have strong inhibitions, and aggress only when instigation (anger arousal) is sufficiently intense to overcome inhibition. They are therefore expected to attack others rarely, but with extreme intensity if they do so' (Blackburn 1993, p. 238); undercontrolled offenders, on the other hand, have weak inhibitions and aggress more readily and consistently.

These then, are some very brief outlines of the distal antecedents that may contribute towards the development of aggressive tendencies in individuals. However, we also need to sketch out some more proximal factors that may be correlated with violence.

Proximal factors

Proximal factors are those contributory events to aggression and violence that occur immediately preceding the outburst, or at the time of its occurrence.

Environmental factors

The first area of proximal antecedents we would like to consider is environmental factors. This area has received much research investment although much of it remains speculative. For example, changes in the Earth's electromagnetic field resulting from the gravitational forces of the lunar cycle have been said to be responsible for aggression and violence (Lieber & Sherin 1972); however, other studies could find no significant relationship (Mason 1997a). Environmental noise levels have also been studied in relation to aggression and Mueller (1983) has suggested that a relationship exists. Similarly, climatic factors such as temperature have also been suggested to be related to human aggression (Anderson 1989), as have ozone levels (Rotten & Frey 1985). However, Anderson (1989) noted that this relationship could well be accounted for by misattribution by the individuals concerned, and Blackburn (1993) tempers the strength of this relationship by suggesting that these climatic factors may merely alter individuals' rate of social interaction, which governs the opportunities for aggression and violence. Gerlock & Solomons (1983) found no significant relationship between aggression and violence, as evidenced by seclusion rates, and barometric pressure readings, biorhythms or birth signs.

The invasion of personal space (proxemic behaviour) is said to raise anger levels (O'Neil et al 1979) and aggressive persons are said to prefer greater personal space distances (Kinzel 1979). However, proxemic preferences are culturally different, can change over time, with experiences, and differ between individuals.

Substance abuse

The second area of proximal antecedents refers to substance abuse. Alcohol and drugs are popularly held to be related to violence and aggression. We can distinguish three aspects to this relationship: (a) violence that occurs because of the effects of these substances, (b) violence that occurs to support the acquisition and distribution of these substances and, (c) violence that occurs to support that addiction. Although high rates of alcohol use in those who have committed violent offences have been reported in the literature (Mayhew, Elliott & Dowds 1989), no causal relationship has been established. Theories of alcohol-related aggression include disinhibition theories, in which a relationship is said to exist between the effect of alcohol on the brain and the person's lack of control. However, this is too simplistic an argument; after studying cognition in alcohol-related violence, Pernanen (1991) argued that there was a narrowing of the perceptual field that created a more limited choice of behaviours for the person. The situation is further complicated by theories that involve an analysis of the motive for drinking; in these, reduction of anxiety and tension and the regaining of feelings of power are said to be driving forces. Furthermore, other theories have related personality factors such as hostility, impulsivity and dominance to alcohol use and violence (Buickhuisen et al 1988) but, again, these theories are contradicted to some effect by the findings of placebo and antiplacebo studies (Bushman & Cooper 1990). Likewise, with drug-related violence there are contrasting research findings and the great difficulty in controlling for personality factors and situation factors makes it difficult to conclude that there is any firm relationship. Lack of distinction between violence caused by the drug itself and violence undertaken to acquire money to purchase the drug is also a confounding factor.

Cultural and situational factors

Finally, the way in which people view themselves in relation to their cultural group is also said to influence their tendency towards violence. Zimbardo (1970) suggested that levels of anonymity are related to violence and factors such as the extent to which a person is involved in their cultural group, and the feelings of felt responsibility spread across members, contribute to a condition of *deindividuation*. This condition involves a loss of self-esteem, decreased self-awareness and an unconcern for consequences, which make the person more likely to respond to aggressive cues. There are also studies that suggest that the victim plays a part in precipitating the violence enacted against him. Wolfgang's (1957) suggestion that the majority of homicides were triggered by the victim being the first to resort to aggression led to a negative response from some quarters and the claim that this suggestion 'blames the victim'. More recently, however, it has also been reported that violence occurs owing to retaliation following insults (Felson & Steadman 1983) and also in an attempt to save face (Berkowitz 1986).

In conclusion, we can see that violence and aggression occur in a complex dynamic that involves the aggressor, the victim, the environment, the situation and the culture in which it is set.

DYNAMIC CONSTRUCTS OF VIOLENCE

As we began to explore in Chapter 1, the major consideration of violence in any given society is the level of appropriateness of its use within cultural and contextual rules of engagement. Actual levels of violence considered appropriate can range widely, from an acceptable level of assertiveness in maintaining one's position in a queue to extreme levels of raw violence in defence of one's life. However, there is also the question of degree of violence employed within a given context.

Historically, when violence was made manifest, and visible, for those actively engaged in attack or defence, it was usually a question of survival. However, in contemporary times, for most people, the violence in our society is no longer this primordial question of survival, and the remnants of this savagery and terror are sublimated to other mediums of expression. This elementary fear is periodically unlocked by the horror story and the violent video, although in these cases it is tempered by the safe distance of the narrative within the book or the film. It can be turned off, and turned away from, at any moment of choice. Furthermore, the fear that is evoked is sheltered by its being 'unreal', at least unreal in the sense of it being rooted on the page or screen. When the fear that it elicits becomes too uncomfortable it can be tamed by this notion of 'unreal' and can be located as mere fancy, fantasy or fabrication. Even true stories are merely stories being told. However, when violence and fear are made 'real', they form a dangerousness that becomes more tangible. Dangerousness then moves from being evoked by a perception of violence that has its place *inside* the imagination to a place now situated *outside* in the reality of someone's behaviour. It becomes concrete and corporeal, and thus has the potential to create pain and threaten our well-being. This appears as much the case in psychiatric settings that deal with violent persons as it does on the football terraces. When violence is thus made visible, it tends to jar on the sensitivities of those observing on the periphery, and reverberates a dormant chord in their primal psyche. This chord is composed of the fear of vulnerability, weakness, injury, pain and death.

Nowadays, as members of society, we generally encounter violence from the distance of fiction or the TV documentary or the news. However, when we are conscious of it occurring for real and within our vicinity, in our 'lifeworld' as Schutz (1970) would call it, the feelings that it engenders become more intense. For example, when we see a brawl in which one person is getting seriously injured by another person, there is a tendency for us to feel a range of emotions, which contribute towards what can be described as a profound empathy. This is based in our own fear, anxiety and dread of becoming the victim. If we intervene on the victim's behalf, it is in the hope that someone will, in turn, become the rescuer for us. The violence that exists for real, but at a short distance, is a concern to us, as it might lead to our involvement, and thus put us under threat.

However, the violence that lurks at a short distance may suddenly focus on those observing as a new quarry; it then becomes an impending threat that evokes defensive strategies. As the danger becomes imminent, we become cognisant of a state of risk requiring evasive or protective action. This is the moment of crisis when fight or flight are our primeval options. In this intricate dynamic, which holds the structures of fear and its practical concerns, lies the operational repertoire of both lay members of society and professionals working in the field of mental health. As we reluctantly become embroiled in the violent scene, we are forced to commit ourselves to specific courses of action, which can be passive or active, and it is these different options available to us that form the focus of this book. Located in this dynamic of the violent scene, and our roles as spectator, rescuer or victim, lie our choice of actions. These actions are underpinned by societal values and norms in relation to violence, and the defence against, or management of it. This provides the legitimation for such action.

VALUES

Values are complicated social concepts. Each society, group, or subgroup, from a macropopulace such as Western society to a microassociation such as a street gang, have shared values that are standards of behaviour regarded as legitimate and binding for that community. They are social laws by means of which the ends of action are selected, and members of those groups bear allegiance to them. They inform us as to what courses of action in our behaviour are acceptable and unacceptable. Values differ among societies and groups and can be a source of considerable conflict, from major disputes to minor disagreements. Interestingly, they may also be held theoretically, but not maintained in practice (e.g. fidelity may be valued socially, but infidelity often occurs). They are closely linked to norms or what is often collectively called 'normative behaviour'. Norms are prescriptions for human behaviour and serve as guidelines for action. Group living ensures that there are expectations regarding our behaviour and norms regulate our adherence to these rules. As Abercrombie, Hill and Turner (1994) put it: 'Since the term refers to social expectations about correct or proper behaviour, norms imply the presence of legitimacy, consent and prescription' (p. 288). We can now see that these two social concepts of values and norms are closely related to ethics as a system of morality and rules governing behaviour in any given society. What should be borne in mind, however, is that values and norms are not fixed entities but are instead dynamic, that is, they change within societies over time, and this can result in disagreement within a society. What is of central concern to us, here, is the extent of disagreement that exists between mental health professionals in relation to the management of violence and aggression.

The manifestations of violence and aggression are so diverse and prevalent in our society, that values and norms relating to correct behaviour in response to them, are also extremely wide and varied. For instance, whereas killing someone who is about to kill us is considered legitimate as a self-defence strategy, the same action would not be considered an appropriate response to being threatened by a 'road rage' incident. The difference lies in the degree of force required to defend oneself, which in our law should be the minimum required. However, not only is the 'minimum required' a value judgement, but there may be serious consequences to using both too much force, and not enough. This aspect of the dynamic of violence and aggression relates to the social context of the setting; for example, defending oneself in a brawl in a public bar is contextually different to defending oneself against a confused old lady in a bus queue.

Furthermore, when the violence and aggression occur within the context of an organisation that deals with these behaviours as part of its professional repertoire, then the values and norms of the organisational philosophy are also contributing factors in the choice of actions. For example, the armed forces, the police, security guards, psychiatric workers, and staff in children's homes, homes for the elderly and schools, may all have to deal with violence and aggression at one level or another and respond appropriately in context. It is significant that all these institutions have been criticised in the past for inappropriate use of force in managing violence and aggression with their own contextual frameworks.

Within liberal societies, there is a duality of social expectations relating to violence and aggression. The first part of this dualism involves the notion that an individual has the right not to be harmed by another, whilst the second involves the belief that agencies and individuals engaged in control of violent and aggressive persons should not use excessive force in the exercise of their duty. These values prescribe our normative behaviour towards violence and aggression, whether it involves teachers or parents, public or police. This focuses attention on the issues of human and civil rights as we cannot, either as individuals or organisations, be overzealous in our response, as we are accountable to the wider values within human and civil rights legislation. Therefore, these factors influence the repertoire of responses available to us when managing violent encounters. They are part of the expanding dynamic of violence and aggression. We now need to locate this dynamic in terms of a contemporary analysis of modern violence.

CONTEMPORARY VIOLENCE

There is a popularly held view that violence and aggression in our community is on the increase and that our contemporary society is more violent than at any other period in our history. Furthermore, we now have quantitative data that clearly show an overall increase in crime, particularly violent crimes and sexual offences. However, this is too simplistic an explanation as other factors need to be taken into consideration.

For example, history shows that crime in society has been relatively stable for any one society at that particular time. Marsh (1994) points out that we can trace back through history and identify periods in which that society appeared to be in dread of some new wave of violence. In the UK, we had the 'mods' and 'rockers', in the 1960s the 'teddy boys' in the 1950s, and the football rowdyism in the 1920s. In the interwar years society was plagued by 'razor gangs' and in Victorian times we had the 'garotters', who engaged in violent robbery involving choking the victim to death (Marsh 1994).

Also, statistics on crime may merely reflect a greater sophistication in how information is collected. Clearly, if more offences are drawn into a data-gathering process, then this may swell the rates. There are also the 'dark figures' of crime – that is, unreported offences such as sexual attacks, unrecorded crime in which only cautions may be made, and undetected criminal activity, which simply no one is aware of, except the criminal. Yet the popular notion remains that our community is becoming ever more dangerous. Therefore, we need to examine some of the factors that contribute to this idea.

The first point to note is that the *communication* of violence and aggression in society is more thorough today than at any other period. The media of TV news, radio, newspapers, the Internet and World Wide Web, etc. are more rapid in communicating information today than at any other time in history, and are also more encompassing, as the majority of households have TV, and an increasing number are acquiring computers. Therefore, sensational violence is now more quickly broadcast across the country and in some cases, around the world.

Secondly, *expectations* in society have risen considerably with the expansion of capitalism. The emphasis is upon achievement and acquisition, in terms not only of material possessions, but also of status symbols, lifestyles and other signs of success. Furthermore, we can see that there is an expectation that the state should provide for us in times of hardship, which creates a dependency on the welfare state. The expansion of capitalism has not eradicated the class divisions in society and may well have widened the gap. As members of the underclass fail to achieve and acquire to the same degree as peers within their group, their failure may well prompt them to seek an outlet in violent crime.

The third factor we wish to outline is the *relationship* of violence and aggression to other variables in contemporary society. For example, there is a commonly held lay view that mental illness is related to violent behaviour despite scientific evidence disputing this idea (Taylor 1985). Mentally ill people cause alarm in those not used to dealing with them, as sometimes, their behaviour is unusual, loud or apparently irrational. Also, substance abuse (alcohol, illicit drugs, glue, etc.) tends to be linked to violence in the mind of the public, as users often appear 'out of control' and needing to satisfy an addiction. Let us therefore look a little more closely at each of these, as they are examples of the existence of a dichotomy between lay notions and professional understanding.

The evidence for a relationship between mental illness and violent behaviour remains contentious. Hafner & Boker (1982) found schizophrenics to be in greater number in their mentally ill violent group compared with a non-violent group. However, Taylor (1982) found that the violent schizophrenics in her study were aggressive with family members and acquaintances rather than with strangers. Similarly, some authors of inpatient studies suggest that violence is greater in the mentally ill population (Noble & Rogers 1989) whilst others have been less convinced (Fottrell 1980). On the question of alcohol, Coid (1982) suggested that this was probably not related to violence, whereas Bushman & Cooper (1990) claimed it probably was. Goldstein (1989) argued that illicit drugs are not related to violence, whereas Nurco et al (1985) had previously reported high rates of drug-related offending. Clearly, in all these accounts, the evidence for a relationship between violence and mental illness, or substance abuse, remains tentative. Yet despite this, there remains an image among lay members of society that such a relationship does exist, and furthermore, that the majority of mentally ill people are dangerous. It is this 'image' that is of central concern in the perpetuation of this myth.

The image is popularly reinforced by TV and film. Often a murderer or serial killer will be depicted as 'crazed' (i.e. psychotic or psychopathic). Although the majority of studies on TV/film effects on violent behaviour are also inconclusive, the repeated coupling of these images serves to fortify the perception described above. We will return to this image in the next chapter but before we leave it here, it is important to stress that the perception of this relationship, however accurate or inaccurate, does not make it any less real or unreal for the person who perceives it. This image of danger will affect the behaviour of the person and influence the social context in which it is grounded. If these contexts are health care settings then the image affecting our action will also influence our professional behaviour.

VIOLENCE IN HEALTH CARE SETTINGS

The dynamic of violence in health care settings is similar in many ways to that of violence met in social life. However, it appears to have two differences. The first is that those on the receiving end of violence and aggression are restricted in their responses to actions acceptable within professional codes of conduct. This ensures that reactions are confined to standards that have been, by consensus, accepted as those that are legal and utilise a minimum of required force. Although they offer a benchmark by which actions can be judged, they do limit the professional worker's behaviour under a moment of intense stress, which adds a dimension to the dynamic of violence and aggression. However, this is countered to some degree by a second feature, namely the anticipation of support. In health care settings, one can expect that other staff can be summoned in times of crisis to help in the resolution of violent situations; in general social life, this aid is often absent as strangers tend to be reluctant to become involved and professional help in the form of the police often arrives too late. However, we should also note here that the support expected in health care settings can be variable in terms of response time, of poor quality when it arrives, and is sometimes absent altogether. We will return to this in Chapter 5.

Irrespective of this difference, we should be aware that the fear and danger that are felt in response to any violence and aggression, are very real indeed. The only qualification to this is that, whereas one person within an encounter may perceive a high level of danger and feel a great deal of fear as a result, another person within the same encounter may perceive a lower level of danger with a resultant lower degree of fear. Furthermore, someone else may not perceive any danger at all, or feel any fear whatsoever. This latter situation can occur because previous similar encounters may have produced experience of safe resolutions contributing to a stock of knowledge by which other encounters are judged. Or it may merely be, that no cues were comprehended during the encounter.

Just as violence and aggression are seen in all societies, and can occur in all walks of life, they can and do arise in all health care settings. They can be seen in children with autism, with learning difficulties, or with behavioural disorders whilst they are at home, in school, or as inpatients. Adolescents in hostels and homes can become violent and aggressive for many reasons, from engaging in substance abuse to responding to peer group pressure. Adults arriving in accident and emergency departments, intoxicated by drink or drugs, can be extremely difficult to manage, as can sober adults suffering frustration from long waiting times, grief at loss of a loved one, or anger at a perceived perpetrator also attending casualty. Often elderly, confused and demented patients in hospital or nursing homes can become violent, and although their frailty limits the extent of danger, none the less, their aggression may cause injury. Anger is not restricted to patients, as relatives and visitors can also become aggressive for any number of reasons.

CONCLUSIONS

As we have begun to explore, in this chapter, the theories and antecedents of aggression and violence, we note that these can be far reaching and complex. This is also the case in clinical terms in health care settings, where aggression can range from the violence seen in some toxic confusional states to the aggression seen in some postepileptic fugues. Sometimes violence is manifested by patients suffering from brain trauma, recovering from anaesthesia, or in postsurgical psychosis. Some mentally ill persons and those with personality disorders may be violent and housed in psychiatric hospitals, secure units, special hospitals, or in hospital wings of prisons. Thus, we can see that the range of theories accounting for violence and aggression is extensive, the number of possible antecedents is vast, the types of clinical conditions are considerable, and the health care settings are diverse. As we have pointed out, it is important to understand these conceptual underpinnings in the management of violence and aggression, as they may lead to effective treatment. For example, a person who has a brain tumour may become aggressive and surgery may remove the tumour, which results in eradication of the aggression. However, in this book we are more concerned with the management of violence and aggression as it comes closer to us and ultimately embroils us in the physical effort of practical management. We are concerned with the encroachment of violence and aggression in the developing encounter, the eventual crisis and beyond, rather than in the long-term therapeutic management. Therefore, we turn our attention in the next chapter to the phases of the encounter and the cycle of aggression that can develop.

3

Phases of violence and the aggression cycle

KEY POINTS

1. Violence and aggression are social phenomena.
2. They have become psychiatrised concepts.
3. This creates a tension between lay experience and professional practice when managing violence and aggression.
4. We can draw on both lay and professional domains in the practical management of violence.
5. There are models available that focus on the role of fear in staff and patients in establishing cycles of aggression.
6. There are phases of aggression during which a deterioration is noted and interventions may be applied.

INTRODUCTION

In Chapter 2, we began to identify some of the major theoretical studies on violence and aggression. We distinguished between theories of aggression and those of antecedents, and set out distal and proximal factors that may contribute to the exhibition of violence and aggression. We noted that most violence and aggression occur within a social matrix that inevitably involves others, that this dynamic differs from society to society, and may also differ among community subgroups. We also debated the wide-ranging social structures that form our image of violence and aggression, including TV, film and literature, and then discussed the social values that govern our response to actual violence. Reviewing contemporary violence, we have argued that the popular notion that violence is on the increase in our society, was not as clear-cut as it seems. However, it is clear that the communication of violence has certainly become more comprehensive with present-day technological advances. This has contributed to the idea that all mentally ill persons are dangerous and that all extremely violent persons are 'mad'. Finally at the end of Chapter 2, we discussed the differences between the dynamic of violence and aggression in health care settings and that occurring in general life.

We now wish to turn our attention to the management of violence and aggression from an organisational perspective. First we will discuss briefly the rise of mental health care settings whose primary goal is the control and management of violence, founded upon medicalisation of the dangerous individual. We will then analyse the role of health care professions in the management of violence and aggression, from both an institutional and a community perspective, and briefly discuss social organisations such as the police, security firms and the armed forces, where a primary function is the control of violence, often in its extreme form. Medicalisation of individuals has produced a battery of risk assessments for dangerous individuals and these will be briefly sketched; from this we will be able to offer the reader an overview of recent work concerned with establishing the profile of violent and aggressive individuals, although the results to date are mainly inconclusive. We will then go on to illustrate the aggression cycle, outline various factors that maintain it, and offer some suggestions as to how it may be interrupted. A cognitive model for understanding the role of fear, in both staff and patient, will be outlined to show how emotional responses can influence behavioural action. Finally, we will outline the three phases of violence and explore the relationship between each of the stages. Managing violence may involve the use of force, which, in effect, is a form of violence itself. This topic will be elaborated in the conclusion to this chapter.

THE MEDICALISATION OF VIOLENCE

The idea of a relationship between violence and mental disorder has a long and chequered history. Most early accounts of mental aberration involve, to one degree or another, some aspect of violent behaviour occurring during phases of psychiatric crisis (Aurelianus 5th century AD). The depiction of madmen and madwomen chained and fettered in dungeons during the

Dark Ages is well noted. Certainly, the pioneering libertarians, Pinel and Tuke, would have had no one to unchain had these conditions not existed. John Conolly's (1856) treatise on psychiatric treatment without the use of mechanical restraint is testimony to the fact that mechanical restraint was a mainstay of the psychiatric armamentarium of that epoch. There is no suggestion that the violence of deranged people was directly treated, rather, it was merely controlled and confined by the use of restraints. Any 'treatment' was of a secondary nature involving debilitating potions and shock caused by any number of contraptions. The mechanical restraints to which Conolly referred were, literally, chains and manacles, which he replaced with moral imperatives and seclusion for disturbed behaviour.

To understand how the medicalisation of violence occurred, we need to relate it to the psychiatrisation of the dangerous individual. According to Foucault (1978) the 'dangerous individual' became medicalised during a 35 year period between 1799 and 1835 in Western Europe. This occurred as courts of law began to be persuaded by psychiatric testimony in serious cases of murder or extremes of violence. The psychiatrists of the time were able to convince the courts by describing a clinical condition known as *homicidal monomania,* which was later realised to be fictitious. This condition was portrayed as a rare, but violent, occurrence that caused the afflicted person to act in a criminal way; thus the dangerous individual became the province of psychiatry, after which, it fell to those working in this field to apply a 'treatment' and effect a 'cure'.

Just as the theory of homicidal monomania allowed 'dangerousness' to become the domain of psychiatry, so to, did the developing theories of violence and aggression (highlighted in Chapter 2) permit these to become medicalised concepts. The comprehensive and complex theoretical explanations of violence and aggression suggest that they are responsive to 'treatment' at the hands of the appropriate expert. In consequence, violence is now a supposed area of expertise for many mental health professionals. However, this idea may well be as fictitious as that of homicidal monomania 200 years ago. Moving the focus of management of violence and aggression away from control to treatment, has shifted the emphasis from technological to psychological approaches. However, this has had its drawbacks. Staff finding themselves in a face-to-face encounter who respond by attempting psychological techniques are at risk if aggression leads to an assault. Furthermore, once an attack occurs, it becomes necessary to resort to means of control, at least in the first instance, as a means of self-defence.

There is a commonly held view that the reforms undertaken at York, in Britain, and the Saltpetre, in France, were designed to offer a greater degree of liberty to the patients, and most assuredly, the unfettering of manacled patients was a laudable enterprise in anyone's view. However, as Foucault (1967) observed, it was not totally libertarian, as a system of morality was applied and a compliance with the rules was expected and anticipated. For example, patients were expected to work and to contribute towards their keep. They were also required to comply with the doctor's orders and succumb to their will. So the application of morality was merely another form of restraint. Similarly, in contemporary treatment of violence and aggression, there is an element of moral imperative applied to patients to get them to develop self-controlling measures. This can take the form of an assessment of their internal control formation, their response to identified cues, and their extent of victim empathy.

What has become apparent is that within the notion of the medicalisation of violence and aggression in which mental health professionals work, there currently exists a dichotomy between psychological treatments, within the morality of liberty, and technological control, within the morality of self-defence.

THE GROWTH OF EXPERTISE

Violence to another person is such a fundamental threat to the well-being of both the individual who is likely to become a victim, and the social fabric of the community, that the response to it has generated a massive growth industry. To circumscribe violence and aggression, using systems of containment as well as systems of treatment, a variety of different organisations have developed to fulfil specific social roles. The police force maintains law and order but is often also at the frontline in managing violence and aggression. Members of the police have also been trained in basic skills in identifying psychopathology in offenders and suspects to ensure early and appropriate referral to mental health services, and are also able, under the Mental Health Act (HMSO 1983), to transport a suspected mentally ill person from the community to a place of safety. Legislation allows for the compulsory detention of those considered to be a danger to others; the police, lawyers and courts may seek a psychiatric referral when members of the public are apprehended or brought before them, if they consider that their actions may be the result of a mental disorder, or that they have a mental disorder that results in them not being responsible for their actions. Thus, much of society's structures have developed to protect its members from harm caused by others, and it is no surprise that fundamental aspects of religious teaching, education in schools, and parental guidance are based on the principle of not doing harm to others.

Social institutions, such as the police, armed forces and security firms have developed response strategies for the management of violence specific to the context in which they are likely to meet it. For example, whilst members of the armed forces may well learn how to kill in defence or attack, one would not expect a private security firm to engage in similar activity; this latter group would learn evasive techniques for defensive and protective purposes. It is not only the context in which violence is met that differs, but also the levels of it. This is an important point to remember when considering the options available in its management in health care settings. In dealing with violence in the community, different groups have developed specific areas of expertise. For example, community psychiatric nurses are often concerned with patients in society who may cause harm to others, as are probation officers with offenders on licence. Similarly, social workers have clients who are deemed a danger to others, as well as those who are victims of violence. Thus each group represents a body of expertise concerned with the circumscription and control of dangerous, violent, individuals in the community, and this control has been legitimated through legislation and professionalisation.

This growth industry also includes the development of institutions who manage, to one degree or another, violent persons. Prisons contain a number of people who act violently in society and, since these people may continue to harm others whilst incarcerated, prison management has firm policies, practices and procedures, as well as training, to deal with violent offenders, to safeguard both other prisoners and prison staff. Special hospitals cater for dangerous, mentally disordered, offenders who are often violent and aggressive, and have developed specific expertise in their management. Medium and regional secure units and clinics also manage mentally disordered offenders requiring lesser levels of security and serve the community through their own referral system, transferring patients to and from special hospitals. Numerous other specialist units and psychiatric facilities also continue to manage violent persons but can likewise transfer extremely difficult patients to secure establishments. All organisations have contributed to a growing body of practical knowledge and expertise in the management of violence and aggression.

Historically, the expertise has not been generally shared, but merely passed on through generations of employees within individual institutions. However, there are a few authors who have contributed to the development of institutions for the management of violence and aggression with practical recommendations, both on the large and on the small scale. For example, MacCulloch & Bailey (1991) discussed the issues in the provision of forensic services from a macro perspective whilst Craig Ray & Hix (1989) offered architectural plans for a suite of secure rooms to manage violent individuals. The expertise that is more readily shared is the academic work on the assessment and management of risk in relation to dangerous violent persons within both the criminal justice system and the mental health system.

RISK MANAGEMENT AND THE ASSESSMENT OF 'DANGEROUSNESS'

Although the concept of 'dangerousness' is understood in the literature to refer to the propensity of the patient to reoffend when released back to the community, it overlaps considerably with the behaviour of the person within the health care setting. The clinical assessment of dangerousness must deal with two major problems: the first is that of assessing a patient as dangerous when in fact they may not be, and the second is one of assessing a patient as not dangerous when in consequence, they are able to go on to assault. It is only when mental health professionals are *wrong* in their assessment that it becomes of central concern. However, this situation is likely to occur clinically as mental health professionals are statistically less than 50% accurate, tending towards overprediction of dangerousness (Monahan 1984).

However, the longer-term prediction of dangerousness is not the focus of this book but rather, it is the short-term prediction and management of violence and aggression. Although it is recognised that short-term violence constitutes a criterion for the longer-term assessment of dangerousness, the immediate concern for those dealing with short-term violence is that those likely to be performing the assessment are also likely to be the victims should they get the assessment wrong. It is this closeness to the violence that establishes an urgency in striving for an accurate prediction of long-term dangerousness from the occurrence of short-term violence. Clearly, knowing the previous history of the person is important in this scenario.

Categorical rating of dangerousness

Marra, Konzelman & Giles (1987) attempted to assess dangerousness using a combination of an investigative approach followed by a categorical rating. In their method, an evaluation of a patient's records is made using the patient's psychosocial, medical and legal history as a primary database. This is then compared with known correlates of violence established from previous behaviour patterns that have resulted in dangerous behaviours to produce a possible future prediction for the patient in question. The patient is then given a low-, medium- or high-risk marker. Patients may be rated on the categories of: history of dangerous behaviour, institutional records, stressors and means to violence, victim and environmental factors, mental disorder, psychological testing, actuarial scales and other moderating factors, to give a graphic representation of their dangerousness. Marra, Konzelman & Giles (1987) stated that: 'the result is a profile that represents the complex interactions of these ratings and the ability of the clinician to visually assess consistency' (p. 295).

Statistical approaches

There are other approaches to the assessment of dangerousness. For example, Harris, Rice & Quinsey (1993) developed a statistical prediction instrument derived and validated from a group of serious offenders. They included many subelements within the broad headings of childhood history, adult adjustments, index offence, and assessment results. These authors concluded that this instrument significantly predicted violent outcomes (Harris, Rice & Quinsey 1993). However, these types of statistical approaches are viewed unfavourably by nursing staff on psychiatric units who tend to believe that they, themselves, are more likely to predict dangerousness.

Lambert, Cartor & Walker (1985) studied ratings of nursing staff on almost 700 inpatients using, in the first part of their study, the care 10 form, and in the second part, a more general analysis of item variance with computerised mathematical models. They reported that: 'nursing reports of dangerousness were unreliable. Even ratings of staff actions, such as "emergency action in the last 30 days" were mostly erroneous' (Lambert, Cartor & Walke 1985, p. 39). Another method recently developed is the Crisis Triage Rating Scale (CTRS) for psychiatric emergencies (Turner & Turner 1991), a scale that builds on earlier work that determined whether or not admission to hospital was necessary. Although the CTRS has also been used for the purpose of assessing need for admission, the important development for the management of violence and aggression was the addition of subscales to measure dangerousness, support systems available and the ability to cooperate. There is supporting evidence of the predictive validity of the CTRS (Turner & Turner 1991) yet, despite this, the ability to predict violence within health care settings remains relatively neglected.

One study assessing the clinical judgement of violent behaviour in the short term was that of Kirk (1989). This study included 68 patients who were compulsorily detained in a locked mental health detention facility. Legal papers were reviewed to determine admission criteria and information gathered on the patient on an ongoing basis. Violent behaviour was rated on both verbal and physical aggression scales. The results failed to 'show a significant difference in the incidence of violent behaviour between detainees judged to be a danger to others and those judged not to be a danger to others' (Kirk 1989, p.349).

Tanke & Yesavage (1985) analysed 12 assaultive patients who had provided visible cues of violence and 13 patients who had not. Using a number of factor analyses, they developed subscales in: thinking disorder, withdrawal–retardation, anxiety–depression, hostility–suspicion, and activation. Using these, they found that: 'the two sub-group populations of violent patients appeared to differ from one another with respect to characteristics of psychopathology' (Tanke & Yesavage 1985). Their general conclusions were that there was a distinction between high and low visibility of potentially violent patients, primarily in the hostility–suspicion and withdrawal scales. However, it should be noted, of course, that psychiatric nurses tend to intervene in high-visibility violent patients to prevent them from attack and therefore, not surprisingly, they are the focus of closest attention.

All the above require, to some level, that a certain amount of history pertaining to the aggressive person is known. When this is the case and a past history is available then making predictions is easier, although no more accurate, as we have noted. Two important points, which will be explored more fully later, are as follows. Firstly, sometimes we have little or no previous knowledge of the aggressive individual concerned, as the situational encounter may be an emergency room, admission unit or a casualty department. This calls for an assessment of what the situation entails and what options are available at that point in time only. Secondly, although we may not have much information on this violent person before us, we do have available a 'stock of knowledge' gained from all other previous encounters. This is a rich source of both our successes and failures of action in previous violent scenes and can be drawn on in our current evaluation.

PROFILES OF VIOLENT AND AGGRESSIVE PATIENTS

It should be stated at the outset that anyone can become violent and aggressive given the right set of circumstances. In this section, we therefore give a broad overview of studies that have attempted to provide evidence of a relationship between violence and a given number of variables.

Colson et al (1986) studied 127 psychiatric patients who were considered violent in the long term and extremely difficult to treat. They readily accepted that the term 'difficult to treat' can cover an array of problems manifested by a diverse population in many differing contexts. They therefore subdivided the broad category of 'difficult to treat' into: (a) withdrawn psychoticism, (b) severe character pathology, (c) suicidal–depressed, and (d) violence–agitation. It is the last grouping which we focus upon here. The authors reported that the diagnostic category in this group included a high proportion of schizophrenic disorders, the highest rankings for total incidents and also a requirement for more special controls than the other groups. An interesting finding was that the profiling of these patients by factor analysis revealed 10 subcategories of which, violent agitation was the fourth most difficult to manage. The authors also reported that profile (a) (the most difficult to manage) was a pansymptomatic group, which comprised: 'three men and three women with various diagnoses, two major affective disorders, three with "other psychoses", and one with a personality disorder' (p. 722).

Sex

There have been some attempts to relate assaultive behaviour to various personal characteristics of the violent individual. For example, males have often been associated with higher rates of violence than females (Evenson et al 1974, Garai 1970). However, there have also been studies reporting higher rates amongst females than males (Fottrell 1980) and others recording no significant difference (Hodgkinson, Mclvor & Phillips 1985, Tardiff 1981). Furthermore, Tardiff & Sweillam (1982) noted that although 65% of their sample were males, when the sample was subdivided according to age it was revealed that the majority of assaultive patients were under 25 years old and predominantly female. The reverse was the case in the older age group (26 to retirement age). Haller & Deluty (1988) suggested that, according to Feschbach (1970),' as females get older, aggression is more likely to be inhibited and to become a source of conflict. While early aggression in females is subsequently inhibited during the socialisation process, in males, such behaviour is often regarded as sex-appropriate and is, therefore, sanctioned' (Haller & Deluty 1988, p. 176).

Age

Age ranges have also been studied in relation to aggression and violence; there is a general consensus that the occurrence is greater in the younger age band (Fottrell 1980, Shader, Jackson & Hartmatz 1977). However, some studies have reported no significant relationship between age and assaultive behaviour (Tanke & Yesavage 1985) while still others report higher rates in both a younger group (20–29 years of age) and an older group (60–69 years of age) (Hodgkinson, Mclvor & Phillips 1985). Explanations for the general trend for violence to reduce, the older one becomes, are related to the general slowing down and physical weakening of the body, as well as a change in appreciation of one's vulnerability and susceptibility to injury. The increased rate of aggression in the older age band of 60–69 years of age in the 1985 study of Hodgkinson, Mclvor & Phillips was that this group was largely made up of psychogeriatric patients with dementing illnesses.

Clinical diagnosis

Assaultiveness has also been studied in relation to clinical diagnosis. Schizophrenia has been recorded as accounting for most assaults (Pearson, Wilmot & Padi 1986, Tardiff & Sweillam 1982). However, some studies include categorisations that are too broad for meaningful interpretation. For example, Lion, Snyder & Merrill (1981) reported their 'acutely psychotic' group as accounting for the majority of assaults; whilst there may be differences between acute and chronic, and between psychotic and non-psychotic, the extensiveness of such categories makes it too difficult to draw firm conclusions. 'Character disorder' was reported as responsible for the majority of assaults in Ionno's (1983) study, which again includes a variety of diagnoses.

This diversity of reports of diagnostic categories reflects a fundamental bias in the manner in which studies are undertaken. Data collection and analysis require rigorous applications; otherwise a particular group of patients may be described as responsible for the majority of assaults, without comparisons being made with non-assaultive patients in the same diagnostic categories. This was eloquently highlighted by Haller & Deluty (1988) who argued that 'a major problem with most of the studies is that the primary diagnoses of the *non-assaultive* patient in each sample were not assessed or reported. Discovering that most of the assaultive patients in a particular sample are diagnosed schizophrenic is of very little value if most of the non-assaultive patients in that sample are also diagnosed as schizophrenic' (p. 175).

Race

Despite the great concern about racial discrimination and prejudiced practices in psychiatry, there is a paucity of empirical studies of aggression according to race. However, this is not to say that no such work has been carried out. Tardiff & Sweillam (1982) found that most of the assaultive patients in their study were white, but this contrasts with the earlier report of Allon (1971) that suggested that blacks are more disturbed than whites in relation to the type of diagnosis. Some authors report a racial bias, for example: 'black patients, however, are over represented on all types of Mental Health Act sections; not only from the police but those signed by general practitioners, psychiatrists and courts; for each this over representation is of a similar order' (Littlewood & Lipsedge 1989). However, other authors found no such racial bias (Tanke & Yesavage 1985).

Experience of nursing staff

The grade and experience of nursing staff have also been examined in relation to the violence of patients. These studies begin to explore the concept of the motivation for aggression being a social entity, rather than simply something inherent within the aggressor – that is, the aggressor and victim may be intricately involved in a self-fulfilling prophecy of social disharmony resulting in eventual combat. Although some studies have suggested that younger, inexperienced staff are more likely to be the victim of assault, there is also evidence that a complex relationship exists between professional grades, age and attitudes of staff (Hodgkinson, Mclvor & Phillips 1985), as more experienced staff are likely targets of violence, but that there are also peaks with both first and second level nurses.

Health care setting

Understandably, the context in which violence and aggression occurs has also been studied. The results suggest broadly that psychiatric intensive care areas, high-dependency areas and admission wards have systematically reported higher rates of aggression (Fottrell 1980, Lion, Snyder & Merrill 1981). This, of course, is not surprising given that the more disturbed patients tend to require these facilities. However, other areas of hospital care recording high rates of aggression and violence, include psychogeriatric wards (Hodgkinson, Mclvor & Phillips 1985), casualty departments (COHSE 1977) and forensic units (Coldwell & Naismith 1989). What all these areas share in common is the presence of people with an increased level of disinhibitedness that manifests itself into violence in one degree or another. Other factors studied include the daily events occurring within health care settings; for example, Ionno (1983) reported that violence on visiting days was more common. Some studies have reported increased aggression in the mornings (Dooley 1986) whilst others have recorded evening as a peak violent time (Coldwell & Naismith 1989). In most psychiatric settings, the periods of peak nursing activity, such as meal times and medication rounds, have also been reported to be related to increased incidence of violence (COHSE 1977, Mason 1995). One study has reported higher rates of violence on wards with a 'reduced structure' (Edwards & Reid 1983). By this it is assumed that the authors were referring to the rigidity of boundaries set by staff and the extent to which rules and regulations were arranged and enforced.

The context is also closely associated with the wider cultural matrix of mental health care settings; this involves those sets of beliefs, ideas, prejudices, concepts and ideologies that govern our everyday thinking (Billig et al 1988). Within the mental health care settings that focus on the management of violence and aggression, there are two models that are of specific relevance to the practicality of managing violent scenes. We will continue by looking at these in some detail.

MODELS

The aggression cycle

Presenting a paradigm for understanding and managing cycles of aggression, Maier et al (1987) offered an interactive model that takes as much account of the role of the staff in the sequence of events, as it does of that of the aggressor. Furthermore, it incorporates the function of the administration in supporting the management of violence and addresses the overall relationship of fear, anxiety and countertransference in the cycle of violence. From the numerous models on offer in the literature, the reason why we have selected this one foremost is that it treats each contributing factor of the cycle in an objective manner rather than subjectively denigrating personal feelings to a subordinate level. This is important as a central aspect of this cycle is the fear that violence generates in all concerned and it is in this fear that we ground our own ideas. Let us now look at the 'cycle' a little more closely (Fig. 3.1).

This model of the physical aggression cycle is concerned with how a situation of violence and aggression can occur in which each factor and action can become locked into a self-fulfilling circuit constantly reinforcing itself. With overt-physical violence, where the danger is imminent, the staff response is usually quick and 'take-down' is usually initiated, which involves physical restraint. Where the danger is not imminent, then 'talk-down' is usually attempted, which involves talking the person out of further aggressive action. According to Maier and his coworkers, the threat to the staff in facing a 'take-down' situation is different from that in a 'talk-down' situation. During the phase of verbal threat of aggression, the stress that is felt by staff members can be chronic, extended over long periods and highly internalised; it is not often shared, talked about or discussed in any forum. Such internalised feelings of fear become insidiously dangerous and can result in countertransference of negative emotions towards the aggressive person. On the other hand, 'take-down' situations usually result from actual violence occurring, which demands immediate action and in some ways relieves the stress of working with long-term threat. Staff are usually supportive towards each other and rapidly respond to ensure a show of force. However, although following a 'take-down', staff spontaneously enquire about any injuries that may have been sustained, rarely do they ask about feelings of fear.

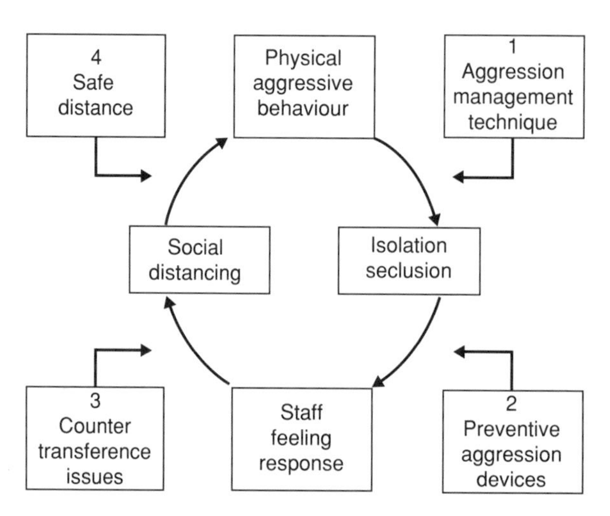

Figure 3.1 The physical aggression cycle. (From Maier et al 1987, in Hospital and Community Psychiatry, vol. 38, p. 521. Copyright 1987, the American Psychiatric Association. Reprinted by permission.)

The aggression cycle has several features. Firstly, there is the physically aggressive behaviour itself, which requires some form of intervention. Secondly, interventions may be of several types: isolation, medication or physical restraints. Thirdly, the staff develop negative feelings about the patient and, fourthly, social distancing occurs as a result of countertransference. Finally, this social distancing reinforces the physically aggressive behaviour and increases the likelihood of violence reoccurring.

The authors set out nine points designed to counteract this self-reinforcing circuit; they included an increase in nursing staff, redesign of their training programme, the development of preventive aggression devices, and the establishment of 'me-times' in which staff discuss their own feelings in response to aggression.

What is important, for the present discussion, in this model, is that although it results from studying a unit that specialises in the management of aggressive individuals, of a somewhat chronic nature, it incorporates items that are highly relevant to acute settings. Irrespective of whether one meets aggression on a regular basis, or relatively rarely, the feelings of fear induced, cause staff to alter their behaviour toward patients. Furthermore, when a situation of aggression is met in the future, it triggers the memory of the previous assault and contributes to the choice of reaction, whether positive or negative.

A cognitive model

A second model that we wish to consider here is the cognitive model of seclusion as a stress-coping strategy, which was developed by Whittington & Mason (1995) (Fig. 3.2). This model was developed specifically in relation to the use of seclusion as a response to violence, but the conceptual framework within which it is located is relevant to all violent encounters.

The model is based on the level of threat perceived by the person who is assessing the situation. This is a cognitive process whereby the appraiser categorises a situation in relation to the harm that could be done to her well-being. The two central questions in this evaluation are 'Am I in trouble?' and 'What can I do about it?' (Folkman & Lazarus 1988). There are two possible answers to the first question: (a) 'The situation is "irrelevant" or benign-positive' and (b) 'The situation is endangering, or challenging, to me'. As far as facing violent persons is concerned, the first answer is unlikely to occur. The second is far more likely, and in this scenario, there will be an emotional reaction from the person under threat. This emotional response can range from low to high intensity and will govern how we act in the situation. Although the cognitive model suffers somewhat from circularity, it is useful in focusing again upon the role that fear plays in the management of violent encounters.

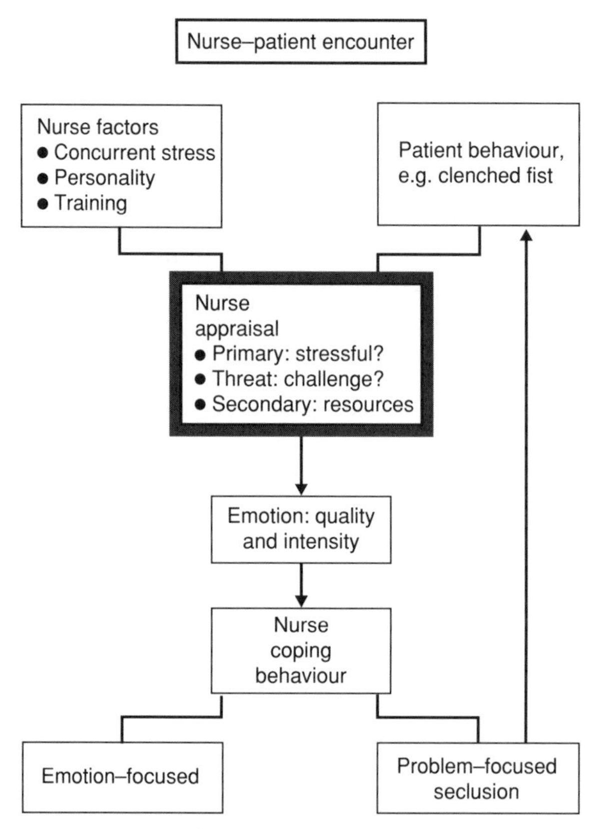

Figure 3.2 A cognitive model of seclusion as a stress-coping strategy (based on Folkman & Lazarus 1988). (From Figure 1, Whittington & Mason 1995, Journal of Forensic Psychiatry, vol. 6(2), p. 293, with permission of Routledge.)

Both the above models are grounded in the human response to perceived threat and both suggest that the options available to persons in this scenario are very much rooted in this fear. We now need to look more closely at a violent encounter and the phases of management that accompany it.

PHASES OF VIOLENCE AND AGGRESSION

The events leading to the crisis of combat, including balancing judgements appropriately, deciding on interventions, and evaluating the situation accordingly, are challenges that face most clinicians who manage violence and aggression. Moreover, the responsibility for taking decisions at any stage in the 'decision tree' confers a heavy burden, considering the potential consequences when things go wrong, as they sometimes do. It is therefore useful to practitioners to focus upon the repertoire of possible responses in intervening in a deteriorating situation to prevent actual violence.

The events of violence and aggression can be divided into three distinct phases. They are observable in the majority of cases of violent outbursts and form useful stages for organising options available at any given time. Although we have clearly delineated these phases, it should be emphasised that the actual boundaries are, in practice, often blurred. Notwithstanding this, it would appear that the margins become more clearly defined with the developing experience of individual clinicians. As always, however, an element of personal interpretation is inevitable in most violent cases, as we need to draw on experiences in our social life, as well as in our professional domain.

Figure 3.3 refers to the perceived stages of deterioration towards a crisis that involves violence. These are represented as phases 1, 2 and 3.

Phase 1

Phase 1 indicates an area of activity that is a relatively normal state of affairs. For those who are being treated for their history of violence and aggression, it includes the entire repertoire of therapeutic activities. For those mental health professionals working with violent persons, this is the phase in which everyday therapeutic activity occurs and is potentially a valuable area for a variety of interventions. In non-psychiatric settings, this phase would involve an awareness of the potential for violence but an appreciation that at this point in time the violence is dormant. What is important in this first phase is the concept of *awareness*.

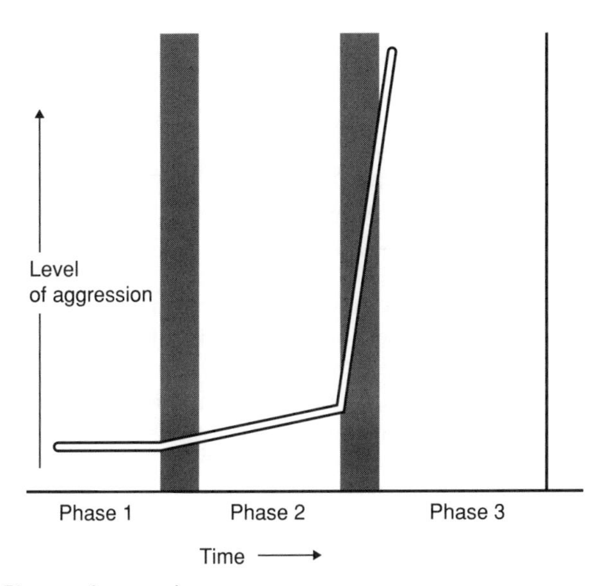

Figure 3.3 Phases of aggression.

Phase 2

Phase 2 is a preaggressive stage when prodromal signs and symptoms of a deteriorating situation are generally evident, but no actual violence has occurred. This stage may include intuitive interpretations regarding a general unease in the 'atmosphere'. Those involved are usually aware that something is wrong, although it is often difficult to define exactly what that something is. For instance, a tenseness is often noted, either in oneself, other professionals, or patients. It is important to understand that in this phase, there is an abundance of options available for intervention.

Phase 3

Phase 3 is the loss of control and the emergence of actual violence requiring some form of physical restraint. In this period, the person engages in combat and is non-responsive to verbal intervention. The options available are diminished at this point.

Boundaries between the phases

As was mentioned above, in practice, the boundaries between the phases are blurred, but with experience, they become more focused. The boundary between phase 1 and phase 2 can be defined as that moment when there is an awareness of a change in the relative normality and when one should begin to scrutinise the situation more closely. Successful interventions at this stage can divert the aggression and return the situation to a 'phase 1' state. Many violent outbursts are prevented here and anyone working with aggressive individuals will readily recount such interventions. These generally go unnoticed by others and probably do not get recorded as events. There is usually plenty of time to deal with events at this boundary, as cues are still being noted regarding a possible deterioration. The deterioration may occur within an individual person who is becoming more disturbed and manifestly more aggressive, or it may occur in a dynamic between two or more people. In any event, the correct intervention is required to interrupt the development to phase 2 and reinstate phase 1.

The boundary between phase 2 and phase 3 is different. At this junction, time is usually of the essence. The move to actual assault tends to be explosive with the person lashing out, throwing something, or smashing furniture. There is little time to peruse the options available; the options have in any event now become more limited. This is a dangerous situation for all concerned and appropriate action is needed swiftly. Although we represent the boundary in Figure 3.3 by two sets of fixed lines, in reality, it may be more abrupt than this and our awareness of the move to phase 3 may actually be triggered by being attacked ourselves, witnessing an assault on others, or hearing an alarm. The form that the violence takes will dictate, to some degree, which of the now limited options are adopted. For instance, if a person is destroying property it may be prudent to allow him to dispense some energy on this before physically intervening, but this must be weighed against the increased opportunity for acquisition of weapons (e.g. broken glass). On the other hand, if a person is physically attacking another person, then an intervention is needed immediately.

Levels of aggression

Finally, we would point out that on Figure 3.3 the x and y axes representing the levels of aggression against time are also not set entities. The level of aggression in each phase varies with the individual assessor and the slope of the line through each phase has been drawn quite arbitrarily. In an individual case, the line through phase 2 may be sharper and more inclined, or shallower. Similarly, the span of time in each phase may be more protracted or shortened, depending again on the individual and the situation.

Before we move on, we would point out here, again, that the long-term therapeutic management techniques involved in phase 1 is not the focus of this book, with but rather the options available in phases 2 and 3. These phases are dealt with in more detail in subsequent chapters.

VIOLENCE ON VIOLENCE

The words 'violence' and 'aggression', as we pointed out in Chapter 1, have negative connotations and we tend to view them distastefully. However, again, as mentioned earlier, a certain amount of aggression is needed to function in society. What we wish to focus on here is that some level of violence may be necessary to overcome the violence of others, although, because of its negative undertones, we feel compelled not to use the word violence but to employ the term 'force' instead. Someone gently escorting a disturbed person to another area of the ward may, in some cases, need to place a friendly hand on the person's arm, or while applying mechanical restraints, may need to use a degree of force, and certainly will most assuredly need to use some restraining force while struggling with a combative person. However, in all these circumstances, the motivation for the use of force is based on certain assumptions, firstly, that the force used is the minimum required, secondly that it is a benevolent act and thirdly, that it is controlled.

Much of the physical management of violence and aggression is now formally attended to in training and educational programmes, which may be provided by in-service departments or external agencies. However, despite the assumptions of 'minimum required force', 'benevolence', and 'controlled', none the less, as far as the recipient is concerned, it may well be perceived merely as violence and aggression undertaken by staff – as indeed, at one level, it is. Therefore there should always be a dialogue with the patient at the appropriate time about the actions that necessitated the use of force by staff.

CONCLUSIONS

Violence and aggression are such a fundamental aspect of our society that organisations have developed whose primary function is to safeguard society from dangerous individuals. These organisations include not only the physical structures of prisons and hospitals but also the social structures of police and community workers. Areas of 'expertise' in the management of violence and aggression, which take many forms, have also developed. Of these, risk assessment and risk management are the subjects of huge research activity, as are attempts to identify profiles of violent persons. In the control and management of violence and aggression, there are a number of models to aid our understanding. The aggression cycle model shows how a self-reinforcing circuit that involves both staff and patients can be established. Similarly, the cognitive model highlights the role of perceived threat in facing the violent encounter. The phases of violence and aggression have been identified and interventive options in their management can be located within these phases. Finally, it is realised that the control of outbreaks of violence requires some element of force, which can be interpreted by recipients as violence and aggression undertaken by staff.

In this first part of the book we have focused on the theoretical underpinning of the management of violence and aggression, and we will draw on this in Section 2. The theory of violence is important as it can contribute to the practical management of aggression but it should also be noted that the majority of people also have a large corpus of knowledge available to them from their own social world, and this can be drawn on in the management of violence and aggression. In Section 2 of the book, we will turn our attention to the practical aspects of controlling violence and aggression as the violent encounter comes ever closer.

SECTION 2

Options available in the phases of violence and aggression

SECTION CONTENTS

PHASE 1

Phase of relative normality

4

Observational, surveillance and diversionary techniques

KEY POINTS

1. Observation is a critical element of managing aggression.
2. Both recognised psychiatric and lay signs can be indicative of a preagressive phase.
3. Technological surveillance can help limit aggression and alert staff to potential dangers.
4. Diversionary techniques are often the first attempt at avoiding violence.
5. Verbally de-escalating hostility is often achievable, and more desirable, than physical intervention.

INTRODUCTION

The hostile encounter is never a pleasant experience although it is fair to say that its effective management may well be rewarding. As we have mentioned earlier, the perception of violence and aggression precipitates a hormonal response that prepares the person for either fight or flight. However, for those charged with a duty of care, neither of these two options, in their literal sense, are acceptable. What is required, instead, is a controlled response using well-tried and tested formats based on accurate observations. Situations are often effectively managed before they reach the physical stage by a combination of learned professional skills, manipulation of resources, and experience inherited from the staff's social worlds. It is clear that the earlier the potential for aggression is recognised and identified as such, the earlier some intervention can be attempted. Clearly, this is preferable for all concerned, as it reduces the possibility of injury and maintains the health and safety of both the aggressor and the victim.

In Section 1, the first three chapters set out the theoretical backdrop to violence and aggression. Whilst this theoretical substance is important, particularly in terms of providing a sound knowledge base informing practice, there is currently an added urgency to provide practical advice. Theory can often seem distant from the realities of managing violence and when you are in the throes of physically attempting to control and manage an aggressive person, it may feel somewhat irrelevant. However, even under such conditions, the theory will inform that practice, which suggests that the theory and practice of managing violence and aggression are conjoined.

In Chapter 3 we saw that in phase 1 there is no indication that a situation is deteriorating towards becoming violent, and that in this phase, the long-term treatment and management of violence are an ongoing endeavour. However, in phase 2 we note a deterioration is perceived, an indication of something changing. At this stage, it may well be merely an intuitive feeling, a hint of something different, or a suspicion of something 'going on'. It is at this moment that observation plays a crucial part, for without it, we cannot progress to further interventions. Following effective observations and surveillance, we may apply a diversionary technique, which could possibly prevent a violent encounter coming to fruition. The present chapter sets out the various forms of observation, surveillance and diversion and shows how each complements the others in the overall management of violence and aggression.

OBSERVATION

Observation is possibly the most singular important action in the management of violence and aggression as it forms the basis from which all interpretation of behaviour is derived; yet rarely do health care professionals mention its importance. People in potentially violent and aggressive situations instinctively feel a need to observe more intensely and those observations will be pivotal in the effective avoidance, control and management of that situation. Observation has six definitions in the concise Oxford English Dictionary (1992), the most pertinent of which are '1 the act or an instant of noticing; the condition of being noticed. 2 perception; the faculty of taking notice.' However, noticing does not sum up the complete activity in terms of the effective application of observation in the present context.

The social dynamic

In any given situation, one clearly needs to know what to look for, which requires an understanding of the context in which the situation is developing. For example, a noisy gang of drunken youths in a hospital's accident and emergency department creates a situational dynamic that requires careful consideration, as does an angry relative in the waiting room. However, we can clearly see that the situations themselves are vastly different. The power of purposeful observation is derived from our knowledge and experience of these various situations, and this includes understanding our own role within the social dynamic. Just as the situation is created by the gang of youths or the angry relative, so too is it developed by our own impact on the scene. We ought to be aware that, although the role of the professional involves attempts to be objective in these difficult situations, subjectivity is often at the forefront because of the presence of fear and trepidation. In managing aggression, the observer and phenomena are intertwined, and pressures to be objective in practice often translate into demands that some theorists would claim are impossible (Clarke 1995). Subjectivity is generally accepted to be an opposite concept to that of objectivity; however, in the present context we may better understand the function of subjectivity if it is defined as a type of bias. As observers, and reporters, of observations, we should therefore seek to reduce this potential bias through understanding the complex relationship between individuals and the social situation that they observe.

It would appear appropriate to recognise the fact that practitioners are a social influence on the health care environment and that their personal histories and presence will affect the context of a developing situation. Subsequent interpretation of a scenario will be based on personal judgements (see Chapter 14). Although personal history is not a justification for any particular interpretation and response, we should be aware that it is an influence on people's perception of the events being studied. For instance, judging of others by one's own ethnocentric norms is always going to be a potential flaw in any professional's practice. This can best be reduced by gaining an awareness of the issues surrounding our own socialised expectations that govern our judgements and actions.

What to observe

Psychology informs us of the difficulties in eyewitness accounts of events. For example, several people witnessing the same car accident may well perceive different aspects of the crash resulting in considerable dispute regarding actual events. Furthermore, in witness testimony, it is usual to request a description of the 'facts' and to avoid interpretations or explanations. However, in the management of violence and aggression, it is precisely the latter that is required in order to attempt assessment and intervention. For this, it is important to examine observational frameworks in order to provide a systematic approach to the assessment of aggressive situations.

Microcues

Within any health care setting containing an individual who may be perceived as potentially causing harm, there are fundamental indicators, known as microcues, that form the basis of the assessment. Dubin (1981) offered four central points of observation that should be given priority in the assessment procedure. These are as follows:

1. Posture – observe how the patient is sitting or standing. If he is sitting tensely on the edge of the chair or is gripping the arm rests, the interviewer should be cautious and alert to the fact that increased tension often precedes violent behaviour. If he is standing, assess whether his posture is aggressive (e.g. hands on hips, leaning forwards, or jabbing a finger in a particular direction).
2. Speech – the patient's speech can be a clue to his degree of agitation. Is he talking in a calm voice, or is his voice loud and strident? Is he verbally threatening? The louder and more strident the patient's voice, the greater is the potential for violence.
3. Motor activity – perhaps the most important and most ignored sign of impending violence is the patient's motor activity. Someone who is unable to sit still, and who paces around, poses the most serious threat of violence.
4. Past history – a past history of violent behaviour is a further clue to predicting violence. If the patient states that he has attacked people before, and at that moment, feels like he wants to attack someone, it should be assumed that he will act on his feelings. At times there is a tendency to overlook verbal threats of violence, but in the context of a past history of violence, a verbal threat is a serious prognostic sign (Dubin 1981).

Stereotyping and prejudice

Drawing on experience from our lay social worlds, we are aware that we often stereotype and generalise incorrectly in our perception of others. For example, if you see a group of heavily tattooed 'skinheads', wearing a type of cut-down uniform, approaching on your side of the street and shouting noisily, it is likely to cause you a degree of alertness or even alarm. Later knowledge that they were, in fact, charity workers on a fancy-dress project, collecting for children's homes, may alter your initial perception. None the less, as social animals, we make such initial judgements on the basis of our own knowledge, experience, attitudes, prejudices and the extent of socialisation. It is important to stress here that in our social world, such judgements may serve to safeguard our social and physical well-being. However, if we were to act on such judgements as the above (and some people do) against such a misperceived threat, then probably, it is we who would be considered aberrant.

An observational framework

In a professional setting, we may usefully employ an observational framework from our social world as long as we are in a position to feed back false perceptions and re-examine our prejudices in light of new information. General observations that may be useful are listed in Box 4.1.

Box 4.1 General observations from the social world

1. Facial expressions
2. Talking loudly
3. Waving arms around
4. Use of bad language (indicator of disinhibition)
5. Alcohol consumption
6. Egotistical
7. Lack of insight
8. Impulsivity
9. Maladapted behaviour
10. Incongruous behaviour
11. Showing unwanted interest
12. Demanding (as opposed to asking)
13. Arrogant behaviour
14. Brash attitude
15. Unusual eye contact (particularly staring or avoidance)

As the situation is more closely observed, the skilled worker can begin to scrutinise the individual more specifically and note the external factors influencing the dynamic more incisively. First, there is a need for an examination of the mental state which those with experience in managing mentally disordered persons can take from their conceptual frameworks. However, those lacking in specific psychiatric expertise may also need to make an assessment of a person's mental state, albeit that this will be limited and somewhat superficial. Again, a reasonable starting position is to draw on personal knowledge of social life and begin to apply a professional framework. The following framework is one example:

- General appearance:
  Is this consistent with the patient's age, gender and social status?
  Does this reflect the patient's cultural group?
- Reaction to others:
  Is the patient hostile to all, some, or specific individuals?
  Is he friendly to anyone?
  How is he reacting to newcomers to the situation?
  Is he fearful, anxious, agitated or aggressive?

- Behavioural pattern:
  Is he consistent in hostile/friendly interactions?
  Is he pacing, looking furtively, or checking around himself?
- Speech pattern:
- Is he rambling, shouting, rational?
  Does he make sense to you?
  Is his voice unusually high/low, fast/slow?
  Is he threatening or abusive?

When making an assessment, the observer should answer these questions and attempt an interpretation by asking what the answers mean. For example, if under speech pattern, the observer answers that the patient is incoherent and slurring his words, then this might be interpreted as that the patient was suffering from drunkenness, drug/substance abuse, head injury, or some form of comatose state, amongst other, possible conditions.

Situational factors

The above leads us to the observation of situational factors that may be contributing to the person's potential for aggression. Clearly, if a patient is further influenced by other factors, then the threat posed can be assessed to be potentially proportionate to the presence of those extra influences. Amongst the most common significant factors that can contribute to aggression are the following:

1. substance abuse or alcohol intoxication
2. substance or alcohol withdrawal
3. acute organic brain syndromes
4. toxic confusional states
5. acute psychotic states
6. paranoid states
7. borderline personality disorders
8. antisocial characteristics
9. head injuries
10. semicomatose states.

Levels and types of observational approach

There are numerous approaches to managing observations of disturbed persons or potentially violent situations; they are as diverse as the clinical areas in which they are set. Many factors will converge to determine the level and type of observation, for example, the role and function of the setting, the amount of support available, the number of staff on duty, the geographical layout, the extent of perceived aggression and the objectives of the observations. However, common themes emerge to provide an overall framework of levels and types of observational approach.

The aims and objectives of the observational approach should be discussed with other staff before undertaking the function, and general factors of concern, if known, should be outlined. Relief changes should also be known and there should be communication of what to do in the event of an incident. Staff must be relieved by another staff member for breaks and should be frequently replaced as observation is a very intensive activity. It is also a stressful endeavour for patients themselves owing to the invasive nature of the technique, and great skill and care are needed to ensure that the situation is not made worse by such close scrutiny. Observational approaches also have an interpersonal and interactive element (see below).

Observational approaches may be classified as follows.

- One-to-one observations – on this level, one staff member is made responsible for accompanying one individual patient wherever the latter goes. The patient is not lost sight of at any time and there are usually restrictions on where he is free to wander.
- Two-to-one observations – this involves two staff members allocated to one patient and usually is employed where there is a raised degree of potential threat by the patient, either to others or to himself.
- Three-to-one observations – again, this is usually employed when the patient is assaultive and swift physical interaction is required to subdue an attack.

In all these levels of observation, staff should be informed as to the proximity to the patient required, which is usually determined by the extent of threat, the expected target of attack, and the objective of the observation. For a further discussion of these levels, the reader is referred to Alty & Mason (1994), Herbel (1990), and Musisi, Wasylenki & Rapp (1989). Other types of observational approaches include:

- Close observations – in which a nominated nurse is expected to know the whereabouts of the patient at all times, although not necessarily accompanying them.
- General observations – which refers to all staff monitoring the overall performance, and whereabouts, of a particular patient.

One good operational account of these types of observational practice is set out in Kingdon & Bakewell (1988). The rationale for such intensive observation is to gain early recognition of clues of potential violence and to formulate a response that will defuse the threat; therefore the quality and quantity of the interactions during the observation period are crucial. However, caution is needed, as the patient can be over-stimulated by constant intrusive questioning and react violently, or may become non-communicative and non-compliant. The approaches by staff members require skilled assessments and careful judgements with well-planned contingencies as situations can change rapidly. Reliance only on qualified staff is a false economy and creates insecurity amongst health care workers such as experienced assistants and aides, who may be equally competent. Unqualified staff members may have considerable ability, irrespective of their professional status. For example, Higgs & Titchen (1995) consider the type of knowledge they possess as being the 'actual competencies required in the field' as opposed to the 'knowledge taught in professional schools' and conclude that outstanding practitioners 'do not have more professional knowledge but more "wisdom", "talent", "intuition", or "artistry"'.

SURVEILLANCE

Surveillance as defined by the Oxford English dictionary (1990) refers to 'close observation, especially of a suspected person'. However, although this definition is appropriate for the monitoring of patients by video in health care settings, it is too narrow for the purposes of this text. Surveillance here means the collection, storage and use of information employed to control violence and aggression by technological means. The amount of surveillance technology employed in social settings has become massive and use of overt systems of, for example, video monitoring in public places is now so commonplace that few give a second thought to it. However, the ethical implications of the use of surveillance techniques are well known and although we may not be overly concerned about being video recorded in the shopping precinct, we would certainly object if the cameras were placed in our homes. Such concerns revolve around issues of privacy and dignity, as well as who is controlling the surveillance, who is doing the monitoring, and what the information is being used for.

We will now review briefly some methods and mechanisms of surveillance that are employed in the management and control of violent and aggressive people. For convenience, they are located under three broad headings of the 'technology of survey', the 'technology of alarm', and the 'technology of control'. However, it should also be noted that there is a degree of overlap between them.

Technology of survey

Most large health care settings now employ some form of closed circuit television (CCTV) system with cameras in strategic positions throughout the unit. Monitors may well be placed in 'hot spots' of potential violence such as entrances and exits, waiting and reception areas, and accident and emergency departments (Drummond, Sparr & Gordon 1989). The advantages of CCTV systems are that they provide panoramic views of the area and give an opportunity to note early signs of any assaults and consequently allow early summoning of assistance. They also provide a record of assaults that is useful in later analysis. The disadvantages of CCTV, however, are numerous; they include a requirement for a constant observer with the inherent problems of distance and boredom, and dislike by staff working in these areas of being video recorded. Molasiotis (1995) noted in CCTV monitoring in health care settings, a complex relationship between the observer, the one-way process of observation, and the discomfort of staff, and found that, although it was a necessary system, the benefits only just outweighed the disadvantages.

The Royal College of Nursing (1994) produced a position statement on the use of CCTV and identified both good and bad aspects to their use. These can be seen in Box 4:2.

Box 4.2 Advantages and disadvantages of CCTV (adapted from Royal College of Nursing 1994)

Advantages	*Disadvantages*
An alternative to locked doors	Patients and their families may object
Patients may have a greater degree of freedom	They are an intrusion into civil rights
They are unobtrusive	They are similar to systems in prisons
They provide more nursing time for patient care	They limit freedom of movement
Reduces serious accidents or incidents	They are less effective in large units/wards
Incidents recorded by CCTV result in less injury	They can lead to reduced staffing ratios
	Nurses are called to aid in incidents

The Royal College of Nursing (1994) argued that the rationale for the use of CCTV was crucial in the decision to employ them and claimed that if they increased patient safety then this was a good justification for their use. Given that violent patients assault not only staff but other patients as well, this may be a point to consider in policy formulation and the use of CCTV. Guidelines for the use of CCTV are rare but we may draw from several sources to identify common themes; these can be seen in Box 4:3.

Box 4.3 Guidelines for the implementation of CCTV (adapted from Royal College of Nursing 1994)

There should be an agreed policy before implementation, which should include discussions with patients, families and interested parties
There should be regular evaluations of their use
Data of incidents should be maintained and reports formulated on successes and failures
Records of CCTV use should be maintained
They should not be used to replace inadequate staffing

Recent research on the use of CCTV would suggest that incidents of assault recorded by video resulted in less injuries than assaults not recorded (Crowner et al 1994a). Whether or not this is because of early intervention is unclear. CCTV recordings have also been used in analysing incidents of assault to arrive at satisfactory descriptions for classifying types of attack (Crowner et al 1994b).

Technology of alarm

Types of alarm system

There are a growing number of alarm systems on the market. These can range from personal alarms carried about the body to electronic alarm systems used throughout units and hospitals. Molasiotis (1995) reported on the use of door alarm systems to control and maintain surveillance of patients who are either confused or agitated, or are combative. However, it should be noted that alarm systems such as panic buttons and door buzzers are only as effective as the staff who must respond to such alarms; this calls for training and clear guidance on policy. Alarm systems for detecting weapons also form a growth industry. Drummond, Sparr & Gordon (1989) reported on the increased use of metal detectors in health care settings to identify those individuals who may possibly be armed. These authors claimed that metal detectors were an efficient and effective technique for discovering potential weapons and offered a defence prior to the intended use of such implements.

Computerised flagging

Drummond, Sparr & Gordon (1989) also reported on the use of a computerised flagging system that indicates the increased probability of an individual patient becoming combative. The electronic flagging system is based on incident report analysis and the notion that 'although prediction of dangerousness is difficult under most circumstances, prediction of repeated violence by a given patient in a given setting may have a higher level of certainty' (Drummond, Sparr & Gordon 1989). Using a computer facility: 'the flag was designed to alert medical staff to the patient's violence potential. When a patient who has been flagged is checked in by a clerk at a computer terminal, or is scheduled for an appointment, an advisory note on the computer monitor appears, and a subtle audio signal is emitted. The flag comprises a brief directive, e.g., "Patient should be searched for weapons", "Hospital police should be asked to stand by until released by examining clinician"' (Drummond, Sparr & Gordon 1989). This provides an early warning system.

Technology of control

The technology of control can involve a wide range of procedures that include the use of one-way mirrors (Musisi, Wasylenki & Rapp 1989), mirrors that are strategically placed to give an all-round view (Molasiotis 1995), and special coded door buzzers (Herbel 1990). However, the technology of control that causes the most contention concerns the electronic tagging of patients.

Removable tags

The use of electronic tags continues, especially for offenders (Davies 1996), despite the complex nature of the ethical considerations and despite the fact that they are costly (Pitt 1987). The tagging of patients who are prone to wander in confusion, and babies in labour wards who may be stolen, is clearly a strategy designed to protect them. However, the tagging of persons considered a danger to others has a different ethical basis. Also, recent trials of tagged offenders in Nottingham, Newcastle and London showed that 40% had removed their tags, which resulted in the offenders being able to go where they should not have been; also the removed tag could be left in an appropriate place by the offender to record erroneously that they were complying with the terms of their parole (Mills 1994).

Non-removable tags

Non-removable tags have recently been suggested to be feasible. Davies (1996) reported this distinct possibility as follows: 'an implant inserted via a twelve gauge needle deep inside the abdomen or neck would be impossible to remove without a surgical operation. A proportion of offenders – particularly first timers – would volunteer for deep implantation if it saved them from the rigours of imprisonment. Given the prevailing attitude to law and order, public opinion is likely to be on the side of the technology' (Davies 1996; pp. 58–9). Although this idea has similarities to that of the control of serious sex offenders through chemical or surgical castration, it is difficult to envisage a time when it would be ethically acceptable.

DIVERSIONARY TECHNIQUES

There are a number of approaches and methods that may be utilised to prevent a person from becoming physically aggressive. Some of these have found their way into the published arena, others are recognised aspects of training packages, with still others remain part of clinical expertise. Successful diversion from physical assault, goes unreported on many occasions, as an incident will have been prevented, and unless these approaches are recorded or researched they will remain unknown to the vast majority, being only part of individual or unit expertise. Furthermore, successful diversion requires a high level of interpersonal skill, which varies significantly between individuals, ensuring that what works for one person may clearly not be the most appropriate method for another. However, common themes and concepts relevant to diversion approaches need to be identified in order to inform professional practice. This section will focus on themes and concepts that can be taken as general principles underscoring clinical and social practice.

Understanding the situation

As we have already noted, many physical assaults are preceded by verbal and non-verbal cues that indicate to the onlooker that all is not normal. These are often perceived by the observer as verbal abuse, angry outbursts, or heated exchanges in which the aggressor is often rude, abusive and sarcastic, or the signs may be more subtle and merely be suspicions aroused in the observational and surveillance stages. However, it is fair to say that when diversion comes to mind, it is usually as a result of an early assessment that a person is about to become aggressive and intervention has to be attempted.

Avoiding escalation of aggression

The first issue to be addressed in diversion involves carers ensuring that they do not become a part of the deteriorating situation by their behaviour contributing to the escalating aggression. If a carer responds to the sarcasm or rudeness in like kind, it is likely only to increase the anger and lead to further heated exchanges, increasing the possibility of overt aggression. If the health worker does become involved in an escalating spiral of abuse, it can lead to a 'Mexican stand-off' situation in which neither party wishes to be seen as the first to back down. One approach aiding the worker to avoid this disastrous possibility is to understand that the patient's verbal abuse and anger may be part of a facade that, in fact, is covering up what the patient perceives as a genuine complaint. Therefore, it is wise to accept some responsibility on behalf of oneself, a colleague, or a unit/hospital with the initial contact, to quietly pose a question to the aggressor, and then, to wait. For example, a nurse may respond to an angry patient with a minor injury kept waiting in a casualty department with, 'I'm sorry that you have been kept waiting', which accepts some responsibility, followed by the question 'I would expect that you feel you have been neglected?' Although the reader may feel that this invites a string of abusive comments, it actually achieves several objectives. Firstly, it 'connects' with the feelings of anger expressed by the patient and suggests that the nurse understands the appropriateness of the anger. Secondly, it offers a chance for the aggressor to reflect upon his feelings by asking himself whether he felt that he had been neglected. Thirdly, it offers both parties a 'breathing space' and the nurse another opportunity to assess the hostility of the patient.

Reducing the tension

The second major issue in diversion techniques is to reduce the tension and not to increase it. Although this sounds obvious, it is often the case that a clumsy initial contact leads to explosive aggression. A good initial contact of 'connecting' with the angry person's feelings by taking some responsibility and then posing a harmless question must be carefully managed by not appearing to be too timid. Do not offer excuses at this stage and do not attempt to lay blame at anyone's door as this tends to exacerbate the anger; this type of exploration is best undertaken much later when the situation has become calmer. Striking the right balance is often difficult; Farrell & Gray (1992) noted that 'offering too submissive a response ... may make patients even angrier if they feel no attempt is being made to understand their needs. Being passive is also unhelpful, and could incite aggression as the patient strives to elicit a response' (p.30). Clearly, one needs to show concern but in a manner that is likely to reduce hostilities rather than make them worse.

Talk-over perspective

Establishing the conditions conducive to talking with a patient who is spiralling towards assault is a skill that requires interpersonal competence in both listening and negotiating (see Chapter 12). There are a number of pointers that can help when engaging a disturbed person in discussion; these can be summarised in Box 4.4 (adapted from the work of Farrell & Gray 1992). The talk-over perspective should be established on an individual basis and according to the assessment of the aggressor's mental state. For example, if a person is clearly rational and lucid, but extremely angry, then open discussion of the events may be the most appropriate response. However, if the aggressor is disorientated, then conversation that distracts him may be more usefully employed.

Averting approaches

We have been able to identify some methods that are best termed 'averting approaches'. Jambunathen & Bellaire (1996) discussed crisis intervention techniques, which are used to reduce the need for physical restraints, and we have adapted their concepts to identify specific strategies to avert a possible violent encounter. These techniques can be usefully applied in the first two phases of the violent encounter (as discussed in Chapter 3

Box 4.4 Establishing talk-over perspective

General principles	*Specific approaches*
Offer support	Do not make retaliatory remarks Reassure the person that you accept that he is angry When the patient make a conciliatory gesture respond accordingly
Ask questions	Ask how the patient is feeling, do not tell him that you know Ask how the situation can be resolved Ask what it is that is causing his anger
Give time	For the patient to think about the situation To review the assessment For answers – do not rush him To hear the full story

above), and are essentially interventions based on human interpersonal contact that are applied to avert impending aggression between two parties. They involve many of the principles discussed in de-escalation, and have as their central theme, the appropriate use of privacy. However, they are additional interventions requiring the health care worker to be socially adept, confident and with the ability to adopt a goal-orientated actor role. The function is to manage the situation away from a perceived audience.

There are a number of requirements for a worker using such approaches. Firstly, he must be able to recognise the deterioration in the social situation and the countdown to a violent encounter. Secondly, the intervention requires that the professional becomes a pivotal interpersonal influence during the decisive moments when the situation is approached. Thirdly, the health worker must place himself at the physical and conversational core of the encounter and become an assertive mediator. Fourthly, the person intervening should remain balanced, equitable and without emotional investment. Fifthly, although the worker's role can change in response to the changing circumstances, at first, commonly, he is in a dominant role and moves into that of the confident benefactor who assists in a resolution. These techniques clearly require skill, confidence and authority, but they can be seen in anyone who attempts, as part of their job, to intervene in an aggressive encounter, for example a referee who attempts to separate fighting rugby players. It is important that the health professional embraces this actor role and carefully manages his voice intonation, volume and pitch, as well as body posture, to convey meaning to those engaged in violence (Musker 1992).

Slow-down approaches

At the point where patients are angry and about to become aggressive and their minds are racing, they are overstimulated and decisions are being made rapidly. In the context of managing violence and aggression, slow-down approaches can help the patient to reduce the speed of decision making (Judge & Millar 1991) and also that of emotional reactions (Gerbi 1994). In practice, slow-down once again uses methods employed by actors, for instance, talking in a slow voice with deeper tone, and using calming gestures to manipulate the responses of the aggressor(s). The approach may also include quietly slowing the pace of situational developments by asking those involved to 'put weapons down' or suggesting 'let's think about this for a minute'. This slows their cognitive pace and helps to begin identifying the issues important to those involved. Physical separation from other patients may be possible at this stage in some circumstances, which not only helps to calm the situation but also removes some people's tendency to perform to an 'audience'.

At this crisis stage, the health worker must maintain as relaxed a position as possible with an apparent casual and relaxed approach whilst attempting to reduce the patient's level of psychomotor activity, the emotional content and the obvious anger. However, caution is needed to avoid appearing ineffective or creating further frustrations by appearing overly laid-back. The balance to be achieved is with being confident, assertive, authoritative firm, and fair.

Verbal de-escalation

These techniques essentially involve the utilisation of the clinician's personal social skills; they are as applicable in managing a potential aggressor in regular life as they are in a worker/patient context. Herbel (1990) stressed verbal intervention rather than self-defence or physical restraints as the first course of action for potentially violent behaviour. This is consistent with the legal position on restraint having to be 'reasonable in the circumstances' (Gostin 1986, HMSO 1993). Clearly, to de-escalate a developing situation verbally is clinically, ethically and legally preferable to using physical restraint. De-escalatory procedures should therefore be utilised in any arena that requires workers to come into contact with a potentially violent individual. Their usage is based on the idea that violence is part of a continuous, usually observable, sequence of events. Essential to the process is the worker's ability to assess safely the appropriateness of approaching combative or assaultive behaviour.

According to Chandley (1995a), 'Verbal de-escalation is a skill based on the theoretical understanding of human stress; and on what nurses refer to as "experience", which implies a degree of insight and the capacity to reflect creatively on past professional experience' (p. 16). Verbal de-escalation is a skilled intervention that is specifically used to intervene when a patient's behaviour moves from being normal for that individual to a state that can be recognised as preaggressive. The technique particularly lends itself to use by health care workers who spend long periods of time with patients, have formed a relationship, and can note the early warning signs. There are three fundamental points to it that are most important, however. Firstly, you must know yourself and be aware of any stressors that are likely to impinge on your own performance. Stevenson (1991) suggests that you should: 'start each day with an assessment of your personal stressors', and should continuously be 'assessing yourself for therapeutic availability'. Secondly, knowing the patient is crucial. Practitioners facing potential violence often comment that management is easier if they have prior knowledge of the patient and his likely responses. Thirdly, it is vital to assess what the patient's needs are, as perceived by the patient himself; as Stevenson (1991) put it: 'determining what the patient feels is needed is critical'.

Listening skills help to validate patients' feelings when they are at a point of frustration and may lead to assault unless defused. These listening skills help the assessor to make judgements about the patient's mental state and give possible diagnostic indications. Chandley (1995b; p. 24) suggests that: 'verbal de-escalation is useful across many diagnostic categories in helping de-fuse situations likely to elicit violence but that the approach to de-escalation changes, qualitatively, depending upon the patient's mental condition'. Leadbetter & Paterson (1995) discuss the concept of de-escalation, which is sometimes referred to as 'defusing' or 'talk-down', concluding: 'that there is no standard approach, and that there cannot be, as every situation demands that a balance of the therapist's social skills be measured according to the exact situation. Any rigidity in approach would render the concept ineffective'. However, general themes are agreed among some authors. Maintenance of respect and dignity is crucial and establishing a trusting relationship is helpful. Furthermore, it is good practice to establish the aggressive situation as private and away from an audience of other patients. Staff behaviour and attitude are important as messages are conveyed both verbally and non-verbally by obvious and less obvious cues that will either diminish or raise the probability of the situation developing into a crisis. Box 4.5 illustrates some of the fundamental requirements for using verbal de-escalation techniques.

Sclafani (1986) also states that verbal intervention has a place in many health care settings and suggests that most 'patients are terrified of losing control and welcome therapeutic efforts to restore control and prevent acting out'. Successful management at this point has many advantages including the prevention of combative behaviour and the minimising of its associated trauma, which both the patient and staff are subject to. Other authors have commented on this type of approach, for example, Philips & Rudestram (1995) suggest: 'maximizing nonviolent outcomes through neutralisation of force and de-escalation of conflict intensity'. Barash (1984) presents the following useful checklist for use at this point to combat crisis.

Box 4.5 De-escalation techniques: practice principles

1. Maintain the patients' self-esteem and dignity
2. Maintain calmness (your own and the patient's)
3. Assess the patient and the situation
4. Identify stressors and stress indicators
5. Respond as early as possible
6. Use a calm, clear tone of voice
7. Invest time
8. Remain honest
9. Establish what the patient considers to be his need
10. Be goal orientated
11. Maintain a large personal space
12. Avoid verbal struggles
13. Give several options
14. Make clear the options
15. Utilise a non-aggressive posture
16. Use genuineness and empathy
17. Attempt to be confidently aware
18. Use verbal, non-verbal and communication skills
19. Be assertive (not aggressive)
20. Assess for personal safety

Do:

- help the patient retain his self-respect by showing you understand his concerns.
- ask how you can help.
- listen carefully and watch for non-verbal signs.
- help the patient to express his anger by eliciting the real issues.
- use reality orientation.
- help the patient to understand his behaviour.
- remind the patient of the consequences of inappropriate behaviour.
- try to get the patient to talk.
- repeat your position.
- offer alternatives.
- use medication.

Do not:

- promise more than you can deliver.
- imply that he will be punished for his anger.
- approach without back-up.
- allow yourself to yell or become aggressive.
- crowd the patient or try to touch him.

Speech patterning

Speech patterning as a means of defusing a spiralling aggressive patient is a recent development that has emanated from work on verbal interpersonal responsiveness (VIR) (Topf 1988). Interpersonal responsiveness is concerned with the degree of expressiveness transmitted when one person interacts with another both through non-verbal means, as well as by the verbal transmission of tone, volume and number of words spoken. Other elements include the extent of intimacy of self-disclosure and characteristics of the manner in which they are stated. Interpersonal responsiveness can be either positive or negative and is an indicator of the status of an interpersonal relationship. VIR lies at the core of human affairs and Topf (1988) has stated that 'many have contended that there is a positive relationship between the existence of appropriate levels of interpersonal responsiveness and success in social situations such as friendship, marriage, work and politics' (p. 9).

The research suggests that there are four aspects to VIR; these are: (a) the number of words used in an utterance, (b) the number of feelings that can be identified through the use of adjectives such as 'happy', 'sad' and 'relaxed', (c) the number of one-word utterances such as 'yes', 'no', 'oh' and 'okay', and (d) the level of intimacy of speech utterances such as self-disclosure statements. The research to date has focused upon the extent of VIR in both staff and patient during an interview situation (Topf 1988). However, possibilities exist for developmental research in this area to identify specific staff skills in attending to such speech patterning, as there are clear indicators that the more socially skilled the staff members are in this area the more effective they will be at defusing the aggressive person.

CONCLUSIONS

In this chapter, we have begun to apply a practical framework to the management of violence and aggression. This was undertaken by offering a framework of observation, surveillance and diversion as the first steps towards achieving this objective. Observation of a situation that appears to be deteriorating towards a violent encounter can be employed using a number of frameworks from both the professional domain and the general social world. However, from both these perspectives, great care is needed to ensure that personal bias is reduced to a minimum before deciding on an intervention. Surveillance has been discussed in relation to the advancement of technology into many areas of life including health care settings; it is an expanding field with possibly serious ethical implications so society will, by necessity, need to tread lightly in order to balance public safety with civil rights. Finally, diversionary techniques have been outlined as the first interventive approach; these include establishing a talk-over perspective, and averting approaches including slow-down methods, verbal de-escalation principles and speech patterning. In the next chapter we will look at the strategies involved in managing resources and the appropriate use of staff in the management of violence and aggression.

5

Resources and staffing

KEY POINTS

1. Resource rationing is a parameter of health and social service provision, and this concept extends to the management of aggression.
2. The environment has a causative relationship to the level of aggression.
3. Environmental manipulation can influence the manifestation of aggression.
4. Positive interpersonal relationships inspire a reduction in the amount of aggression experienced.
5. Staff preparation, training and facilities will contribute to the effective management of violence.
6. Temporal issues including timetables, routines and the ability of the patients to make sense of the time involved in health care are determining factors in the management of aggression.

INTRODUCTION

Chapter 4 focused on the use of specific strategies in the management of violence and aggression; the techniques that were outlined had a base in observational activities. This chapter continues with a form of scrutiny; however, here, attention is turned towards available resources and their subsequent manipulation as preventative factors in violence. Briefly stated, most aspects of the environmental setting can contribute, to one degree or another, to the potential for the expression of aggression. One aspect of the management of violence and aggression is the creation of an awareness that measures can be taken to shape the environment to help prevent violence, control it, and provide a therapeutic milieu for those with aggressive propensities.

An awareness of environmental factors surrounding a potential conflict is important in resolving likely violence whilst minimizing harm to all those involved. It follows, therefore, that once one is aware of the importance of the setting, then clear moves can be taken to manipulate the environment to assist in preventing a crisis occurring, aiding de-escalation, and safeguarding personnel, rather than allowing the environment to contribute to escalating aggression. Much has been said about the need to provide appropriate environments for care, particularly in relation to the opposite demands of, on the one hand, preserving safety and, on the other, safeguarding choice and dignity. Although many health care settings are not built specifically with the idea of managing violence and aggression, it is important that the design of new facilities bears this in mind. Having said that, redesigning facilities can also be undertaken to achieve maximum safety for both staff and patients with the minimum of capital expenditure.

A second resource often referred to in the management of violence and aggression is staffing; this is an expensive resource in financial, personal and moral terms. It often appears that high staffing levels are an aspiration of those who work directly with potentially violent people, but, whilst occasionally it is important to raise staffing levels to maintain safety, it is disputable whether increased staffing always equates with a safer working environment (Morrison 1991). Financial restrictions apply to most contemporary settings, and whilst, in an ideal world the financial budget would provide for the possibility of crises occurring, the actual situation is that unlimited staffing is not readily available. Restrictive budgetary parameters within health and social services have become increasingly inhibiting in recent times and the application of these restrictions to practice areas has resulted in some settings becoming vulnerable. Therefore, how to use available resources in both an effective, and an efficient manner, has become a point of intense deliberation, and sometimes conflict, between service managers and front-line workers. Therefore, it is incumbent on managers and clinical staff alike, to address the provision of human resources for the management of violence within a restrictive financial framework, concentrating on key issues aimed at reducing violence and increasing safe working practices.

The third resource to be considered in this chapter is that of space and time, which are resources that have not received enough attention in the literature. Reducing an animal's geographical space is well known to increase the likelihood of its aggressive behaviour, and human beings are no exception to this fact. Strategies can therefore be employed to ensure that the optimal use of minimal space, through creative and lateral thinking, can contribute to the reduction of tension and the possibility of aggression. Although time is fixed in cosmological terms, its perception can seem to alter as it can pass slowly or quickly depending on activities undertaken. Time in health care settings is often associated with boredom, or with tension and worry, whether for oneself or for another. A lack of activity and information can further compound this experience. Health care staff can help reduce such anxiety through careful consideration of simple factors that patients often feel are of vital importance. This chapter will outline some of these aspects.

THE ENVIRONMENT

Part of the problem in using a term such as 'environment' in relation to the management of violence and aggression lies in the number of variables that constitute its definition. For the purposes of understanding violence in health care settings, the term 'environment' may mean the structure of the building itself, the geographical layout of its rooms, the decor used, the state of disrepair, the space available, the neatness and cleanliness, and so on. It may also include the position of the building in relation to the local community, its location in a wealthy or poor area, whether it is rural or urban, and whether it is easily accessible or not. However, the structure, decor and locale of the building are not the only factors contributing to the 'environment'; others such as the people working in it are also important determinants, for instance their numbers, skills, experience, roles, attitudes, prejudices, etc. Furthermore, their ability to fulfil their function is crucial for the enactment and working of policy, practices, programmes, rules and routines, as well as the manner in which staff time is structured. Finally, the 'environment' includes contributory aspects; among these are the conceptual frameworks used; the philosophy of the organisation, and its individual departments, units and areas; the management of change; and the approach to providing an efficient organisational standard in terms of balancing budgets, resources, care delivery approaches and support for all those patients and staff who come into contact with the organisation. Another general term often used for all these factors is 'milieu'; when viewed as a psychodynamic enterprise, it is often referred to as 'milieu therapy'.

We will now develop each of the above themes under the following headings of 'area design' and 'area organisation'.

Area design

There is much to be said, and certainly much to be researched, about the architectural and interior design of large hospitals, departments, wards, units, clinics and individual areas that cater for violent and aggressive individuals. The importance of establishing the most efficient, productive and safe working practices (MacCulloch & Bailey 1991) in environments that cater for, or are highly likely to contain such individuals, cannot be overstated. However, the factors that contribute to decisions regarding such designs are more likely to be political, economic and personal rather than clinically driven. Thus, we feel it more practical to concentrate on those areas of professional practice that are within the sphere of influence for most practitioners.

The design of individual areas, with the management of violence and aggression in mind, will always be dependent upon the major function of the service being delivered and the extent to which aggressive patients will be seen in relation to the number of patients who would *not* engage in such behaviours. For example, an area that caters specifically for violent persons may require a much more intense and clearer focus of design than would, say, an outpatients clinic that may see violent people only occasionally. A more extreme example would be the design of an admission ward in a high-security psychiatric hospital and a waiting area in an accident and emergency department. Both settings see a good proportion of violence, but in a different context that has to be taken into consideration when designing facilities. However, as is usually the case, certain common themes can be noted, and these are detailed below.

The need for observation

Firstly, areas that accommodate potentially violent situations require some attention to the issue of observations, which was dealt with in the previous chapter. There is little point in organising an area of the unit to contain a potentially violent person if that area cannot be closely observed. Therefore, it is important to ensure that whichever area is likely to be used to receive aggressive persons can be easily and closely observed.

The need for compartmentalisation

Secondly, and in a similar vein, one should attempt to ensure that areas containing such a patient population can be efficiently isolated and secured in the event of an emergency. The area should have the facility of being compartmentalised so that first incidents, and then individuals, can be segregated. This has the added benefit of allowing the business of the units to continue in other areas whilst the situation in the 'trouble spot' is being attended to.

Furniture requirements

Thirdly, furniture is usually required in these areas and careful consideration should be given to it. Areas in which patients are likely to spend only short periods of time clearly require different levels of furnishings from those in which they are going to live for long periods. The provision of furniture also requires attention to the extent of danger that it may pose. For example, in an inpatient area in which patients are going to live for some considerable part of their lives, issues of quality of life may demand that inhabitants have many of the fixtures and furnishings that people have in the comfort of their homes. This may necessitate provision of a lounge area with television, telephone and three-piece suites, because as these are signs of everyday life, they are important symbols of normality and bring with them expectations of appropriate behaviour (more of which we discuss later). In other circumstances, it may be necessary only to provide the basics of a short-term requirement such as seating arrangements. Whatever furnishings are provided, however, one should ensure that: they are robust so that they cannot easily be dismantled for use as weapons, they are heavy or fixed so that they cannot be picked up and thrown, they are inflammable so that they cannot be set alight. It is also worthwhile remembering that furnishings can easily be made into weapons or used as a barricade; therefore this should be borne in mind when developing a unit design (Musisi, Wasylenki & Rapp 1989).

The role of decor

Finally, decor is an important factor that can influence potentially violent individuals. The fundamental decision to be made over decor necessitates an attempt to assess patients' responses to it. One should decide whether to provide a homelike atmosphere that is warm, welcoming and furnished with high-quality material such as curtains, pictures and adornments or whether to equip the area in a more clinical style to give the ambience of a practical hospital approach. In the former alternative, it is hoped that patients will feel themselves to be in an environment like that of their own homes and will therefore behave accordingly, acting with respect and dignity. In the latter, the intention is to produce a clinical environment in which the patient is expected to adopt a sick role and respond to professional health care staff in a respectful manner. In reality, both alternatives often fail in their intention because of the fact that violent people are usually out of control and wish to cause damage. This may be damaging to people, but may also be damaging to property and, indirectly, to the philosophy of care.

Area organisation

It is often the case that health care workers have little opportunity to influence the grand design of health care areas, but they can become involved in influencing minor reorganisation of an existing area. In these circumstances, every opportunity should be taken to maximise the environment in order that violence and aggression are reduced and thus the safety of all is enhanced. Given this opportunity, it is useful to apply a framework that will focus attention and provide a sound rationale for designing changes to existing facilities. We all respond to the environment in which we live and work, and therefore, given the limitations of financial resources, a degree of lateral thinking and inventiveness may need to be employed to achieve objectives. It is useful to consider these under four themes: (a) layout, (b) fixtures, fittings and fabric, (c) extraneous factors and (d) lateral thinking.

Layout

The layout of an area will always be dependent upon the role and function of the unit, the philosophy of its practice and the objectives of its purpose. Observation, so often mentioned before in this book, is a central consideration in area layout. Whether it is of major importance, as in secure settings, or less so, as in other general facilities, it is easy to underestimate the necessity of being able to maintain appropriate observations. Major positioning of areas such as the nurses' station, night station, reception areas, waiting areas, treatment facilities, and administrative sections, is crucially important and these should be situated such that the maximum area under scrutiny can be clearly observed (Warneke 1986). Other areas such as play areas for children, TV rooms, recreation rooms and interview rooms should, wherever possible, be placed around a central, but discrete, observation point. This is important as these areas need to be controlled in the event of an incident.

Fixtures, fittings and fabric

Less major, but equally important in terms of observation, are factors pertaining to the minor structure of area fittings; for instance, fittings such as mobile notice boards should be placed against a solid background and not block areas, corridors or doorways. Another simple, but effective, strategy, is to have mirrors placed innocuously on walls so they reflect otherwise obscured areas.

Wherever possible, furniture should not be allowed to obstruct passageways or doorways, as access may need to be gained quickly. Fixtures, fittings and fabric should always be considered in relation to their potential use in aggressive situations; for instance although a large glass ashtray may be aesthetically pleasing, a small plastic one is more prudent in areas where the potential for violence is high.

As much light as possible should be facilitated to create as bright a setting as is required. Natural light is preferable to artificial illumination wherever possible. If artificial light must be used, then dispersed light against walls, pictures and features is preferable to large banks of fluorescent lighting. However, depending on the function of the unit, this may not be feasible (Geen & O'Neil 1976).

Extraneous factors

Other factors may be, to one degree or another, under our control. For example, noise can be an irritation particularly when it is unwanted and beyond our control. The level of noise of traffic, machinery and the activity of the unit may well be difficult to eradicate but may be reduced by closing windows to traffic, doors to machinery, and addressing civil requests where appropriate to noisy individuals. Other noise such as that from televisions, radios and personal stereos is often helpful in occupying people; however, it can also be extremely provocative to those who do not wish to be disturbed by them. Ventilation is another factor that may be controllable. Hot, humid environments tend to increase irritability and fray tempers; therefore adequate ventilation should be maintained (Geen & O'Neil 1976).

Lateral thinking

The foregoing paragraphs have covered a few basic points, but quite clearly, the number of factors that can contribute to violence and aggression is enormous; in fact, the list is probably endless. Therefore, this section on lateral thinking is included in order to support the creation of ideas, which should be an ongoing endeavour that can provide huge opportunities for ensuring an environment is conducive to reducing the potential for violence. We list a few ideas that have been successfully employed in a wide variety of settings (Box 5.1).

Box 5.1 Some simple lateral-thinking suggestions

Action	*Rationale*
In waiting areas, provide board games, magazines, puzzles, music, television, etc.	Helps prevent boredom and eases the passage of time
Where paintings, tapestries and ornaments are being placed, fix them above head height, preferably out of reach	Helps prevent damage or use as weapons and it raises the head and eyes to prevent ruminating whilst pacing
Sofas and bean bags are better than hard chairs	They are more relaxing
Different areas of a unit should have different decor and themes	Increases interest and distracts from monotony

STAFFING

There is a wealth of literature on the issue of staffing in relation to the management of violence and aggression but there is little consistency in it. There are those who believe that increased staffing is appropriate for managing aggression (Molasiotis 1995), whilst others argue for limiting staff presence (Palmistierna & Wistedt 1995). There are also questions about the best skill mix and gender ratios (Morrison 1990). For instance, although Schwab & Lahmeyer (1979) found no relationship between the age and experience of nursing staff and violent episodes, others have reported a correlation between them (Gerlock & Solomons 1983). The level of experience has also been said to be a correlating factor in the management of violence and aggression; Rasmussen & Levander (1996) noted 'a disproportionately high number of assaults targeted at staff without any formal training'. Lanza et al (1991) recorded that: 'those with less experience may have less skill in avoiding at-risk situations and less clinical skill in handling them' while Bernstein (1981) emphasised that: 'inexperienced therapists were assaulted more often than those with experience of more than 11 years'. In this section we would like to deal with the diversity of problems encountered in managing this issue under two general perspectives: (a) quality versus quantity of staff, and (b) preparation, training and support.

Quality versus quantity

Staffing levels

Fiscal resources and budgetary constraints are a growing concern in every area of health and social service provision as we move into the next century. It is often the case that health care workers, attempting to allay fears and effectively operate therapeutic programmes of activity, will automatically call for an increase in staff as though quantity equates with safety. On the other hand, managers are urged to reduce staffing as they are a high-cost resource and considerable savings can be made by reducing the numbers of personnel. However, the idea of having staffing levels as high as possible to attain safety, is one that has inconclusive support in the literature and is contrary to fiscal reasonableness. The common consensus is that there is an optimum quantity of staffing that a given population requires, but this is not a static measurement, as it changes over time and context. The staffing level, therefore, has to reflect need, and this is essentially something that will fluctuate. The nurse has a clear professional duty to 'report to an appropriate person or authority, having regard to the physical, psychological and social effects on patients and clients, any circumstances in the environment of care which could jeopardise standards of practice' (UKCC 1992). Both staffing levels and staff experience fall within this remit. The measure should be one of whether or not the resources available meet the perceived patient or client requirements (Okin 1985).

Staff qualifications

When one discusses the issue of quality staffing, this should not be confused with the idea that qualification equates with staff quality. This misguided assumption can be an expensive mistake. There are clearly roles that only qualified staff should perform, in line with the guidelines of proportionate responsibility and accountability.

However, often the unqualified personnel are amongst the more effective staff. This group of workers tend to spend more time than others interacting with patients and form a major resource that could often be utilised more efficiently than is generally the case. Unfortunately, poor management tends to dismiss the views, knowledge and experience of non-qualified personnel and minimises them. This treatment appears to be located in the lack of 'legitimacy' of such workers' lay experience and perspective of life as opposed to that in the professional domain. This text argues that, whilst the world as seen through a professional health care view, is of course, considered legitimate, it should not be the case that the alternative lay interpretation, that is conveyed without the accompanying professional discourse, remains unacknowledged. An alternative outlook requires due consideration; this involves a recognition of the value of the non-qualified person's life experience and an awareness that it is important to: 'acknowledge that a major aspect of treating aggressive individuals is based on "art in the trenches" and that over reliance on "textbook theory" can promote blind spots as to what is actually occurring' (Monroe, van Rybroek & Maier 1988).

Interpersonal styles of staff

It follows that if the interpersonal idiosyncrasies of staff can be used to reduce the emergence of aggression and violence, then staff could also, both directly and indirectly, cause an incident of disturbed behaviour. Some interpersonal styles of staff are antagonistic and even hostile, whether they are qualified or unqualified, experienced or inexperienced. Apart from the clear antitherapeutic contribution, the resulting aggression causes undoubted trauma and increases the potential for violence, and whilst this personality type is rare in health professions, the situation when it does occur, must be resolved as quickly as possible. Crowner (1989, p. 109) asserts that: 'interpersonal provocations may be grouped as "noxious stimuli" and considered with the frustration–aggression hypothesis. They are often referred to as "reasons" for assault'. These 'noxious stimuli' can be emitted by staff or patient, and are two factors that will affect a therapeutic environment. Such styles should be corrected to minimise the chances of aggression and to fulfil the duty of care of the health care professional; if this is not achieved, the implications for the patient who is a recipient of this interpersonal style can be quite devastating. As Morrison (1991) observed: 'perhaps the most important finding, and the most controversial, was the importance of the interactional nature of aggression and violent behaviours in persons with a mental illness', which suggests that staff attitudes and dispositions are pivotal in the provision of care.

Preparation, training and support

The preparation of staff in the management of violence and aggression is a statutory requirement under the Management of Health and Safety at Work Regulations, which place the onus of responsibility on employers (Her Majesty's Stationery Office 1992). Staff must be given the required amount of information to enable them to work without there being a threat to their health and safety (Greaves 1994). This preparation includes not only information, but also instruction and training where the risk of violence has been recognised as a problem. Staff will always vary in their abilities, and this is a desirable state of affairs, as some will be more effective at interpersonal skills, others at defusing situations and still others at prevention. However, unless staff receive such information, instruction and training, they will not be fully equipped to maximise their own individual strengths and therefore will be a risk to themselves and possibly also to others.

The preparation and training of staff in the management of violence and aggression can take many forms and will be dependent upon the context in which the health care is being delivered. For example, in settings in which the extremes of violence are anticipated, such as prison hospitals, secure hospitals and intensive psychiatric facilities, training may involve such approaches as C&R, which is a Home Office-approved method of applying physical pressure in the form of strategic holds to control violent persons. Alternatively, in less intense areas, training may involve a more theoretical approach through lectures or open-learning packs. In any event, the training packages now available are extremely diverse, covering most health care contexts, and can be tailored to meet individual needs.

Staff support is often a forgotten aspect of providing a service in the management of violence and aggression, although to be fair, some authors do identify it as a central component (Braithwaite 1992). Staff who have been threatened with violence, or who have actually been assaulted, can be not only physically injured, but also emotionally and psychologically traumatised. Once physical treatment has been forthcoming, the staff support team should provide resources, facilities and time for a full emotional recovery. These resources are, again, as wide and diverse as the requirements of the individual and are vitally important for the injured staff to regain confidence and rebuild psychological strengths.

SPACE AND TIME

Space and time are both philosophical and psychological concepts that most people have an appreciation of, albeit at differing levels of sophistication.

Concepts of space

An example of the awareness of space is that most people can appreciate the idea of freedom of space and certainly can understand when they feel overcrowded and do not have their usual area in which to function. In fact, for most of our lives we have clearly defined spaces for whatever activity we are undertaking, from the definitive lines of a football pitch to the regulated area of living space. It is not surprising that there are some people who suffer from a phobia of too much open space and others from a phobia of too small an area. Space is also a relative concept that is culturally defined, as in the proxemic behaviour observed in chapter 2. Others who encroach, uninvited, into our space are considered hostile and as a response, we either retreat, if we have somewhere to retreat to, or attempt to repel the intruder. Clearly, this can lead to increased aggression, tension and the possibility of violence (Geen & O'Neil 1976).

Concepts of time

Space is something that we have some control over, in terms of the amount that we occupy and what we put into that space. Time, on the other hand, is somewhat different, as this is set by nature if left to its natural course, both in terms of when we begin our existence and when it comes to an end for us. (Artificial insemination and premature termination of life are different matters). Furthermore, without becoming too metaphysical, the passage of time is set by what is known as the 'cosmological clock' (Zerubavel 1987). For us, this means a revolution of the earth equates with a day and a revolution of the earth around the sun is a year. We subdivide the year into seasons as we divide the day into hours and minutes, and we have no control over the speed of these events. However, there is another form of time that is psychologically derived, which is known as the 'inner duration'. This is time as perceived by our minds and it: (a) does have differing speeds of passage and (b) to some degree can be under our influence. We are all aware that a pleasant experience appears to pass faster than an unpleasant experience. For example, an unpleasant experience filled with apprehension, anxiety and tenseness, such as waiting in the dentist's waiting room, seems to pass extremely slowly. Such an unpleasant experience we wish to hurry by and pass more quickly (Zerubavel 1987). Alternatively, a pleasant experience such as a holiday appears to go by rapidly, in fact too quickly, and we would like to slow down our experience of it. These concepts, then, can have a profound effect, not only on the production of frustrations and tensions leading to aggression but also in terms of their manipulation in attempting to prevent aggression. We will deal with these issues within the format first of how space and time can produce aggression and secondly, how space and time can help prevent aggression.

How space and time can produce aggression

The range of people who become involved with health care is extremely wide and diverse. For example, there are those who attend hospitals and clinics for physical complaints, those who become users of psychiatric facilities and those with learning disabilities who require services. There can be few people who have not used the health services, private or public, at one time or another. However, there are some patients who may not wish to engage the health services but are forced to against their wishes and these patients may be compulsorily detained under the Mental Health Act for this purpose (Her Majesty's Stationery Office 1983).

Loss of control

When patients engage a health service, they usually lose some control over space and time. They are required to be in a place chosen by the service whether this be a waiting room, a clinic or a hospital ward. They will also have to wait for service staff to see them and have little say in how long they must remain. They may be transported between departments and wait again for service staff. In the main, they will be told where to go, how long they must stay and when they can go home. Despite the good reasons for the time structuring, the patients' perception can be that the lack of speed and apparent urgency conveys messages regarding priority and importance, which produces expectations of a negative nature. For inpatients, if attention and treatment arrive slowly, or are apparently non-existent, clear messages appear to be emitted about the dual issues of potential length of stay and the individual's low-priority status.

Lack of stimulation

We have already noted that the duration of an unpleasant experience appears to be longer, and this is equally true for traumatic experiences as for boring ones. It follows, therefore, that a period of tension or boredom in a restricted environment, without the freedom to move away, can be potentially traumatising and lead to the increased probability of raised anger and aggression. Patients who have to wait in low-stimulus environments, possibly in pain, discomfort, fear, tension or worry, with no control over their space or time, are likely to lower their tolerance levels (Geen & O'Neil 1976).

For outpatients attending voluntarily, lack of stimulation can be a traumatic experience; however, for patients who are hospitalised, often against their wishes, not only is the control of space and time severely curtailed, but also, both are programmed for them by others. The construction of routines, rituals and timetables is often aimed at the smooth efficiency of the service, rather than the benefit of individuals and, although some services do take into consideration the views of users, service requirements tend to dominate. This itself, is a source of tension between individuals and services, as health care workers create the timetables. For inpatients whose home is temporarily the hospital or unit, the structure of their time and space often equates with ordering their social lives. As Gibson (1994) put it: 'temporality has an effect on peoples lives, and in turn, people manipulate temporality as a means of social order'. Thus, when patients find tension between how they wish to structure their time and space and how the health services organise these, they may become uncooperative, non-compliant and aggressive. This can develop into the patient being perceived as a problem – that is, the patient is seen as 'challenging' the social order, because he will not operate within timetables that are primarily designed for organisational rhythms and efficiency (shifts, routines, commitments) and which clash with the patient's own natural temporal rhythms.

Temporal benchmarks

From another temporal perspective, and the works of Roth (1963) who studied the hospital 'career' of patients, we can see the importance of the ability of the patient to be able to assess his health progress. There are shared knowledges about what will happen next (movement to another ward, extended privileges, reduced medication, etc.) that the patient uses to assess his headway made over time. Rittman (1993) comments that what is required is: 'an interacting group of people with access to the same body of clues for constructing the norms of a timetable'. In practice, Musisi, Wasylenki & Rapp (1989) note that: 'as patients show improvement, they are allowed to go on "reintegration" visits to the general wards', and that after stabilisation, patients are returned to their referring wards. These are meaningful temporal benchmarks from patients' perspectives. Alternatively, and as an adjunct to this notion, Gibson (1994) suggests that another measurement of the passage of time can be the changes that happen to one's peers, arguing that the assessment of one's own health career must be seen in relation to others. Rittman (1993) also argues that, signposts or benchmarks serve as symbols of the passage from one phase to the next. It is essential that patients are able to share common, recognisable signs of such progress and have the knowledge to be able to operate in a manner that enables them to perceive their advancement.

How space and time can prevent aggression

Space allocation

We are all aware of the importance of space allocation in health service settings, whether it be 'our' chair in a waiting room, locker by a bedside, bed space, or own room. We have a sense of ownership and territoriality that gives us a feeling of belongingness, and of a space that is ours that we may be able to exercise a little control over. The significance of this allocation takes on a meaning and relevance defining us as a person in that setting. Therefore, the importance of providing personal space takes on a major significance in helping to reduce the potential for aggression. Great care is needed to avoid belittling the apparently smaller aspects of space allocation by reducing it, manipulating it, or placing something in it uninvited. If these must be undertaken then try to negotiate rather than dictate, which will allow the patient some control over the issue.

Time managements

Time for patients, in health care contexts, needs to be carefully managed to prevent frustration and boredom. However, this management must be undertaken with great sensitivity. Setting timetables should be done with as much flexibility as is possible, allowing for wide parameters of choice. For example, for inpatients, meal times are often rigidly adhered to, thus offering little choice of when food should be consumed and no flexibility in terms of personal involvement in preparation. Timetables also need to take into consideration patients' views wherever possible, and assumptions about patients' preferences should not be acted upon without consulting them. Major events, in this case during the day, for inpatients are known as temporal markers; they segment time for its easier passage. In terms of the day, these comprise meal times, medicine rounds, visiting times and so on. Although these are important for both staff and patients, wherever possible they should be negotiated.

Progress reports

For patients whose inpatient status is part of a health career trajectory, we must be aware of their need for progress reports on how they are doing. For those in long-term care, it is important for the patients to be able to locate their progress against that of their peers, otherwise an individual's health career trajectory may appear erratic. Without the availability of a discharge date, it is essential that patients are able to share common, recognisable signs of progress and have the information to enable them to move towards advancement. The absence of signs and information causes confusion and tension, so behaviour can become unpredictable and aggression increases. In the absence of therapeutic endeavours, real or imagined, the patient is left in a void, a time-vacuum that is then filled with behaviours to thwart boredom. Although some of these may well be appropriate, sometimes they are aberrant and cause further problems.

Reduction of fear

A final note should be made of health care settings that deal predominantly with violent and aggressive patients. Patients in these settings also become afraid of the violence of other patients. Cohen (1994) highlighted the potential 'terror of living with the threat of unpredictable violence' noting that such fear can lead to increased violence as a pre-emptive effort to protect themselves. Thus, space and time, again, can be employed to reduce such tensions and help reduce the potential for aggression.

CONCLUSIONS

Both society in general, and the health and social services in particular, are preoccupied with the management of resources. The impact on state-operated facilities has been substantial over the past 2 decades. In turn, a primary concern of health initiatives has to be fiscal efficiency and effectiveness of actions. There is an urgency to utilise to the fullest the existing resources in our health settings. However, manipulations in the environment and an awareness of its potential can bring about rewards of less violent behaviour. In the greatest proportion of units that meet with aggression, there is a capacity to improve in this respect. More emphasis is required on environmental design, and it follows that if the initial design does not take account of the literature and the wide variety of expertise available, then valuable recommendations may be disregarded that might have impacted on the ability to assure, first, a safe environment and secondly, an environment that can be used positively to affect the health careers of those who require it. The literature is clear that the issues that affect aggression and violence can be separated into environmental and interpersonal concerns. On that basis, staff are crucial, as their ability through professional knowledge and experience, as well as their wider social background, is fundamental to the prevention of crisis and the resolution of imminent combative behaviours. The impact of timetables, routines and restrictions can have a massive psychological effect that can result in further aggressive episodes. An awareness of timetable issues and a bias toward meeting patients' needs, rather than simply organisational needs, can have impressive returns for both the patient at the centre of the hospitalisation and the staff who are charged with improving the health of the individual.

PHASE 2

Phase of Preaggression

6

Intervention modalities and models

KEYPOINTS

1. As the potential for aggression and violence is perceived as increasing there is an impetus to intervene.
2. Distracting the aggressor from the source or target of his anger is possible with a number of techniques.
3. Behavioural approaches may be adopted to defuse aggression.
4. Anger-reducing skills are important in diminishing the potential for aggression.
5. Theory and practice become one conjoint concept when applying interventive techniques.

INTRODUCTION

In the previous chapter, we discussed how resources could be used effectively to reduce the potential of violence and aggression occurring. Resources include the many and varied environmental factors, staffing factors, and space and time. It is interesting to note that although all these factors may contribute to increasing the potential for violence, they can also be used appropriately to reduce such aggression. Their effect tends to depend upon the degree, and context, in which they are set or employed. For example, too much noise can be an irritant and cause increased tension, but sound used appropriately, say in the form of music, can comfort and distract an angry person. Similarly, too little space and too much empty time can cause tension, whilst increasing space and filling time can reduce it. The important point made in the previous chapter is that the management of violence and aggression in phase 2 relies upon skills, knowledge, intuition, experience and inventiveness. Furthermore, the latter can be founded in both the professional and social worlds.

In this chapter, we continue to be concerned with phase 2, as the situation continues to deteriorate to the extent that it is perceived that unless an intervention is made, a violent encounter is likely to ensue. However, here we set out some formal approaches to the management of violence and aggression to provide a theoretical framework for their practical application. This is important as, unless they are applied, they will merely remain conceptualisations. We would also point out here that the transformation of theory into practice often requires ingenuity since the obstacles and hurdles frequently encountered tend to demotivate all but the most enthusiastic staff. The overcoming of these problems requires innovative approaches and some degree of lateral thinking.

In the first part of this chapter we discuss diverting, distracting and deflecting tactics that are focused on engaging the patient in some specific therapeutic activity. The second section deals with several formal interventive approaches, discussing their strengths and weaknesses and providing some suggestions for their practical application. Although grouped under behavioural approaches, they in fact, in their application involve wider cognitive and psychodynamic perspectives. Finally, the theory–practice divide is briefly discussed in relation to the issues involved in the process of converting theoretical concepts into practical applications at the point of crisis management.

DIVERTING, DISTRACTING AND DEFLECTING

There are many methods and approaches that may be used to deflect potential aggression in individual patients, and they may be employed in the first instance, to occupy someone who may become violent, and secondly, to allow an already aggressive person to 'burn-off' his extant anger. In either case, the methods are as wide and varied as the human imagination will allow. Here we present a few well-recognised approaches.

Physical outlets

Patients who are becoming, or who have become, aggressive will tend to have pent-up energy in the form of tension and anger; unless displaced into more appropriate targets, this will probably be directed towards persons or property. Allowing redirection of aggressive feelings towards a substitute target is well known in both professional and lay circles. The provision of such physical outlets in the management of violence and aggression is, therefore, fundamentally important and requires careful considerations about assessment of individual needs. The expending of physical energy also releases the tension of internal psychic energy and is, thus a complementary approach.

Individual assessments should be made in relation to the following:

1. The age of the patient – younger patients tend to be more physical and enjoy various sporting activities; older patients, on the other hand, may prefer a brisk walk and resent being cajoled into more strenuous physical activity.
2. The ability of the patient – some patients may be too disabled, either because of their illness or from prescribed medication, to engage in strenuous activity. Failure at activities can then produce further frustration and anger.
3. The personal preferences of the patient – the physical activity should reflect the patient's personal choices given the limitations on resources.

Physical diversional activity may involve informal approaches such as table tennis, darts or bowls, or more structured programmes offered in a gymnasium or pool, such as football, weight training and swimming. If the patient's needs are accurately assessed and the appropriate available resource engaged, then physical activity can be an excellent diversionary exercise (Her Majesty's Stationery Office 1990, Special Hospitals Service Authority 1993).

Social activities

Many aggressive incidents can be avoided by distracting the patient from his source of anger. There is evidence to suggest that a person who is angry plans his assault by ruminating on the source of his anger (Topf 1988). During this mental rehearsal phase, frustrations build and the increase in tension becomes too great a burden to bear, with the result that violence occurs. By intervening in this build-up, the tension may be reduced in appropriate ways, rather than being expressed by assault or creating damage. Therefore, there should be an attempt to encourage the person to engage in an activity to refocus the aggressor's attention away from his anger. Furthermore, this should be undertaken as early as possible to optimise its effectiveness.

Social activities are often a forceful intervention in this phase of aggression and, again, can be formal or informal. Formal social activities may be part of a structured programme of recreation-type facilities, such as social clubs, film shows and dances, provided for both inpatient and outpatient services. An aggressive encounter can be avoided if the patient can be encouraged to attend such functions as a diversionary approach in the short term but these also aid social relationship building in the longer term. However, caution is also needed as it would not be appropriate to jeopardise others' safety by allowing a violent patient to join the company of vulnerable persons. A balanced assessment is needed to identify the extent to which the patient may respond positively to the distracting technique or whether the social situation is likely to exacerbate the problem.

Informal social activities can also be employed and these include ad hoc activities that can be undertaken as required. They may be simple distracting games, activities that occupy the person's mind or they may be tasks specifically created to deflect attention away from his anger. The important point to remember is that in these activities, it is the occupation of the person's mind with the involvement of others, either staff or peers, that deflects the anger. Possible activities are wide and varied, but staff should be aware that it is often the extent of creative thinking required that provides the basis for innovative practice.

Many clinicians who operate beyond the traditional boundaries of psychoanalytic or pharmacological approaches believe mental health problems, including violence and aggression, have their roots in the social setting of the patient's cultural formation. Living in society brings its own inherent stresses and conflicts, which can be viewed as being aetiologically related to mental health problems. Social psychiatrists have long argued for this interpretive paradigm and consider that the treatment of patients with such problems can only be realistically undertaken if we address the social aspects that have caused the problems in the first instance. However, it is worth noting that, although living and functioning within a social setting can cause problems, they can also be a great source of strength and belongingness and thus be in themselves curative. Such analyses of social activity inevitably involve the role and function of the patients within that cultural setting. Therefore, it is important not only to assess the functioning of the patient within these social environments, but also to provide feedback for positive behaviour during these intervals.

Recreation

There is a balance required between the provision of structured activity (Her Majesty's Stationery Office 1990) in which a programme is designed with specific objectives in mind, and that of autonomous activity that affords the individual a degree of free choice to act independently. A structured programme should have identifiable aims and objectives and not merely be put together because the contents look interesting. The structure should reflect the client group and be aimed at de-escalating violence whilst providing the basis of assessment and treatment. There should be some choice within the programme and appropriate outlets that provide the patient with opportunities for expression. In some instances, short contact with others, on a frequent basis, is better than long contact time with one other person. Providing some autonomy allows the individual to make choices and informs the patient that he has control over his activities. If this control is appropriately managed, then it is a good indicator of the person's internal control state.

When planning activities, there is also a need to 'marry-up' the individual's abilities with the proposed activity, as inappropriate application can lead to problems. If the tasks are too challenging then failure is likely, which can result in negative feelings, and if not challenging enough, then frustration and boredom can be problematic.

BEHAVIOURAL-TYPE INTERVENTIONS

A number of approaches are used to intervene to prevent violence from occurring; these can be loosely grouped under the heading of 'behavioural approaches'.

Aversive techniques

Aversive techniques are broadly concerned with the use of structured behavioural plans that involve a limited sanction, or unpleasant experience, for the aggressor when he shows undesirable behaviour. This technique was adopted in psychiatry for the treatment of alcoholics whereby the ingestion of alcohol, following classical conditioning, was paired with an aversive stimulus (such as vomiting or electrical shock) so that the ingestion of alcohol produced a negative response. Aversive techniques are, of course, fraught with ethical dilemmas and should only be undertaken both within a multidisciplinary framework and under the guidance of a suitably qualified clinical psychologist. The efficacy of these procedures have also been hotly debated; however, one viewpoint is that 'the very existence of the debate about aversive approaches indicates that they must be effective to some extent. If they were simply ineffectual they would not be used and there would hardly be such concern about the ethical issue' (Chadwick & Kroese 1993, p. 240). Furthermore, it could be argued that the criminal justice system itself is based on an aversive principle in that it is a court of law that prescribes the aversive stimulus. (Although, to be fair, others would counter the latter argument with a question regarding the efficacy of this system.)

Contemporary aversive techniques usually adopt some form of social reaction as a negative stimulus to the aggressor's behaviour. These social reactions require careful consideration and meticulous management in order to ensure that they remain productive and do not become destructive entities. Examples of aversive techniques include Darcy's (1985) reality confrontation in which the aggressor is confronted with the victim of the assault and the confrontation itself is the negative stimulus. The aggressor finds that the anger of the victim is an uncomfortable and distasteful experience that deters future aggression towards others. Other approaches involve the use of a privilege system in which privileges can be awarded for appropriate behaviour but withdrawn for undesirable behaviours (as in a token economy system). Peer disapproval can also be used in which, similar to the system in a therapeutic community, the sanctions to be applied can be decided by the patient's peers. This intensive display of peer disapproval, if carefully managed, is a useful vehicle for the encouragement of appropriate behaviour. However, aversive techniques should be used only with the most treatment – resistant cases. They should be employed according to three key principles:

1. They should be used only if they are the least restrictive option.
2. Treatment outcome should include the significant reduction of the target behaviour that will lead to a safe and liberalising benefit for the patient.
3. They should never be used routinely but always as part of a behavioural programme.

DRO and DRI scheduling

Differential reinforcement of other behaviour (DRO) is a behavioural approach that emphasises the building up of desirable behaviours rather than merely suppressing negative ones. The approach is similar to that of a 'token economy' method in which 'tokens' are given when patients respond in a positive manner rather than emit negative behaviours. These tokens can be exchanged for certain rewards and privileges at a later stage. DRO scheduling can be 'either individually or group based, but the latter is far more widely used and is often associated with "token economy procedures"' (Gudjonsson & Drinkwater 1986), which is a form of operant conditioning that increases the likelihood of the rewarded behaviour reoccurring.

In DRO scheduling for violent behaviour, the individual is positively rewarded when he does not aggress. Time intervals are set and he receives a reward at the end of each violence-free timespan. These time intervals are slowly increased as he successfully completes more and more violence-free timespans (Wong et al 1991). The schedules should have: (a) specifically defined goals and target behaviours, (b) a system of rewards that can be delivered immediately and (c) longer-term rewards that support the desired behaviour. Used correctly, the DRO scheduling approach has 'been shown to be effective in reducing aggressive and destructive behaviour; however, that efficacy may depend on the concurrent use of other response-reduction procedures' (Wong et al 1991, p. 300).

A related scheduling procedure, DRI (differential reinforcement of incompatible behaviour), is concerned with the reinforcement of behavioural responses that cannot be performed at the same time as the undesirable behaviour. In this approach, there is a positive reward for these desirable behavioural actions that are incompatible with violence and aggressive behaviour.

Today–tomorrow behavioural programming

Van Rybroek et al (1988) developed the idea of today–tomorrow behavioural programming; in this approach, patients attain a daily privilege level based solely on their behaviour during one day. Changes are made only on a daily basis so that it is 'today's' behaviours that determine 'tomorrow's' privileges. This behavioural programming is generally integrated with many other approaches to the management of violence and aggression but is central in laying the 'groundwork for helping patients that many people feel are "hopeless" cases or the most "hated", since their aggression is a weapon that naturally pushes away all comers' (Van Rybroek et al 1988, p. 3).

Within the notion of today–tomorrow behavioural programming, the progress towards psychotherapeutic relationship building is all-important and those that devise the actual programme are also the ones who implement it. The main goal of this approach is to provide immediate feedback to patients with regard to their behaviour. It is based on the diversional theory of the management of violence and aggression, which suggests that many acts of violence can be avoided if the patient is aware that his actions have consequences directly related to himself. The programme should identify each target behaviour and define rules, limits, permissible interactions with staff and peers and the extent of participation in the therapeutic programme. Once the definitions are in place, a nought-to five-point rating scale is devised, with each point reflecting the extent to which the above are absent or present. The rater scores each at the end of each shift in relation to the scale, and at the end of a day an overall score is attained, which will determine the following day's privileges.

Van Rybroek et al (1988) identified four privilege levels for this scale; level 4 equates with 90–100 points scored on the schedule, with level 3 being 75–89, level 2 being 60–74, and level 1 being 0–59. The success of the today–tomorrow behavioural programming is dependent upon identifying rewards for the patient that are meaningful for the individual and are sufficiently strong enough to motivate him.

Cognitive–behavioural approaches

Cognitive–behavioural techniques (CBT) have predominated in contemporary work in anger management and aggression therapy. However, treatment approaches tend to focus on continuous work rather than on crisis management, and show some success only in the short term, while longer follow-up studies have yet to be undertaken. The most commonly used approach is Novaco's (1978) anger management programme, previously mentioned, which is concerned with cognitive restructuring and the development of coping skills training. There are three stages to it:

1. Cognitive preparation – in which the patient begins to log his experiences of anger and is encouraged to focus on the nature and functionary role of anger. He is brought to a state of awareness regarding his anger and his self-statements. He reviews anger-eliciting situations and is taught how to discriminate between appropriate and inappropriate anger.
2. Skill acquisition – in this stage, there is an emphasis upon learning the skills of anger management and these will include relaxation training, self-control, reappraising anger-eliciting events, self-reinforcement, employing self-instructions, communication skills and assertion training. These are undertaken through taught procedures, reflexive techniques, modelling and role play.
3. Practice application – the acquired skills are then put into practice through a graded sequence of anger situations that are simulations of real-life events. Responses and reactions are tested and feedback is given. The package itself can either be used with individuals or applied in group formats.

As we mentioned above, there is sufficient evidence that this approach is effective in reducing aggressive behaviour in the short term, and it has been stated that 'its utility in managing disruptive behaviour in institutions seems established' (Blackburn 1993; p. 381). However, CBT used in de-escalatory procedures as a response to impending violence have yet to be clearly formulated. Notwithstanding this, it would appear that, given the centrality of cognitive awareness in therapeutic approaches, particularly in stage 2 above, these skills point to appropriate interventive strategies for health workers. For example, knowing that an aggressive person is probably employing self-instructions to an anger situation, an appropriate intervention may well involve eliciting such a statement to aid in defusing the situation.

There are other CBT such as Stermac's (1986) stress inoculation intervention, which is aimed at a cognitive restructuring of anger conditions, and Goldstein & Glick's (1987) method of social skills training, anger control management and moral education. However, although these are variants on the above theme, they also fundamentally revolve around social skills training, anger management and reappraisal of the situational context.

Anger anxiety control

There are many approaches to anger control that are often related to anxiety management, and these are mainly useful for the longer-term treatment of such problems. For example, Novaco (1975) developed a cognitive–behavioural stress inoculation programme that involves relaxation training, preparation for provocation, preparing for the confrontation, establishing an ability to cope with the state of physiological arousal, and offering of self-rewards in the form of personal statements. This programme is developmental in that it can work through a hierarchy of increasingly more difficult and provocative confrontations. Although we only mention this one approach, there are many others; the majority contain the elements of Novaco's approach, some form of social skills training and a problem-solving aspect. However, these methods tend to focus on the longer-term treatment and not the short-term control and management of violence.

Having said this, many of the constructs of such methods are conceptually important for intervention in the management of violence and aggression at the point of crisis, since they involve reducing the state of anxiety that precedes anger (Gudjonsson & Drinkwater 1986). These constructs can be briefly outlined as follows. Firstly, there is latent response appropriateness in which the aggressor is encouraged to verbalise his thoughts on what his choices are at that point in time. The object of this is to stimulate the person into thinking about alternatives. Secondly, the establishment of eye contact is important to develop interpersonal communication. People who stare away or cannot engage in eye contact tend to be uncomfortable, or unable, to relate to the 'other' within people. Thirdly, facial expressions can reveal much about the inner feelings; for instance, the difference between frowning and smiling is well understood. Mirror imaging is common in facial expressions; a smile usually prompts a smile in return, and so on. Fourthly, voice loudness, again, is a common expression of anger. Getting two parties who are shouting at each other to speak quietly is extremely effective in preventing violence, but is not an easy task. Finally, establishing verbal response repertoires is an important component in calming a tense interaction; the frustration of being unable to articulate an issue or the reasons for one's anger can lead to a sudden explosive attack.

Self-soothing skills

A further aspect of applying an intervention to a situation that is potentially violent concerns the personal feelings of the aggressors in the encounter. In those situations where we have applied a defusing technique and have used interpersonal skills, imagination and assertiveness, we are still reliant upon the aggressor responding to our approaches. Self-soothing is closely related to the notion that the violent-prone person requires the responsive ability to regain internal control. In self-soothing approaches, the patient is encouraged to regain his own interpersonal control through the behaviour of others. Obviously, this entails the interpersonal interaction of, and with others, which emphasises the importance of human contact in the deteriorating encounters seen in phase 2.

In encouraging self-soothing skills, it is important to realise the balance of power that exists at the moment that the intervention is applied. Through an assertive intervention, we may well have gained control in a situation but we also need to be aware of the time when we need to reduce the amount of control and allow the individual concerned to regain some control over himself. Remembering that in Chapter 1, we discussed the human necessity for some degree of assertiveness to survive in society, we should at this point allow the patient to regain some authority, which is deemed self-directed and conducive to the overall defusing of the situation. Such self-control can be encouraged through the modelling of prosocial behaviour in which the staff operate within an appropriate role and immediately reflect to the patient a positive social reward for their appropriate response. Positive regard is an easy concept but one that may be difficult to fulfil in the actual situation; it requires that the aggressive patient is spoken to as an equal and given constant reassurance that he can, and will, regain control. Such comments as '*you* do not need to do this', '*you* can stop this when *you* decide to' and 'we will help *you* to regain control' spoken in a reassuring manner offer the patient some positive choices (Rice et al 1989).

Stress-reducing strategies

Stress reduction is another long-term treatment modality that we would like to consider in terms of its role in avoiding the build-up of tension in the preaggressive phase. Stress arises as a response from perceived traumatic events, which may be non-specific – that is, what is perceived as a traumatic event to one person, may well be an exciting one to another. It emanates from the inability of the perceiver to control the traumatising source and to resist its intrusion into his life events (Horowitz 1986). This produces either denial, in which the inevitability is ignored and preparation for responding is put off, or the manifestation of alternative and often inappropriate responses that may include physical or psychological reactions. Recent work in this area resulted in the now well-accepted recognition that traumatic events can lead to the condition of post-traumatic stress disorder (PTSD) (American Psychiatric Association 1989).

If, in a situation where individuals are heading towards a violent encounter, there is an indication that one or more of the aggressors is acting irrationally, this may well be a response to stress. Signs that may indicate post-traumatic stress disorder include an altered perceptual state, ideational processing, various emotional reactions, physical responses and overactivity (Wykes 1994b; p. 116). However, these are general areas that may contain many varied responses within them. Furthermore, they are also easily differentially diagnosed as symptoms of psychoses.

Intervening in an acute phase of an aggressive encounter when stress is considered a causative factor would include removing the stress if possible.

Unfortunately, the original stress that created the problem is often neither manifestly evident nor in the vicinity. For example, one could not remove the original stress caused by being involved in the Vietnam War for those who are suffering from PTSD as a result.

Two factors are important in the acute stage of stress reduction. The first concerns factors associated with distal stress and involves reassuring the patient that he can regain control over his decisions regarding the stress responses, that guilt and regret are naturally occurring emotions in this state, and that success in coping will result in positive feelings. Also included is support in this situation; reassurance should be given that individuals, friends or organisations are available to support the patient. Secondly, there may be stressors in the vicinity that, whilst not the actual causative elements of the original stress, are exacerbating the stressful situation. These should be removed, or the person removed from them where more appropriate, and if possible.

THEORY AND PRACTICE

The reason for including a short section on theory and practice here is that one engages in a defusing strategy at that point when it is perceived that, unless the intervention works, violence will ensue. Although intervention modalities have a strong pragmatic flavour to them, they are thus underscored by theoretical frameworks, so it is at this juncture that theory and practice appear to merge into one. Each influences the other as a particular theoretical idea is attempted and its practical ramifications are fed back to inform further theoretical ideas. At the point of crisis, such a process often happens at a furious pace, with little time for idle reflection or hypothesis testing, and there are many twists and turns of thought and fine tuning of practice. As we point out in Chapter 14, these moments should not be lost or forgotten but brought to the surface for discussion, research and development.

Many of the theories of defusing techniques have a paucity of empirical research to support them, although it is fair to say that this is growing; instead they are generally advocated according to their intuitive appeal. Although there is nothing wrong with this approach, there is a need to explore and test such assumptions in order to develop practice. Simple theories such as 'getting an angry patient to talk will help prevent aggression', may be understood by the assumption that physical violence and talking do not usually go well together. As Rice et al (1989) put it: 'talking and physical aggression are to some extent incompatible behaviours, and thus simply getting an angry patient to talk – and keep talking – should reduce the likelihood of violence' (p. 127). This is an excellent example of a theoretical framework being derived from clinical practice and, in turn, informing the need for further practical applications in training packages and programmes, etc.

At the point of crisis, emphasis is usually laid upon the pragmatic rather than the theoretic aspect, and this can be a drawback unless it is countered by later raising it in discussion as an issue and addressing it through research and exploration. Most approaches to crisis management that are institutionally driven are limited, and in a concrete situation, there are finite options available (Rice et al 1989). This is understandable given that administrators may well be aware of the legal considerations and resource implications, but they will probably have a limited knowledge of the finer clinical issues. Furthermore, in the absence of coherent theory about crisis intervention, other considerations will hold sway in policy development, so although this is a difficult area on which to focus research, the efforts could be hugely rewarding.

CONCLUSIONS

As a crisis develops, and there is a perception that an intervention is necessary to defuse a potentially violent encounter, there are a number of strategies that may be used by health workers to defuse the situation. Some of these can be viewed as informal approaches based on intuition and clinical experience, whilst others are formal and grounded in research. We have here set out some major distracting and diverting approaches, including the supply and encouragement of physical outlets and social activities. Structured programmes of recreation with appropriate outlets for anger management have also been identified and the balance of autonomous behaviour highlighted. Behavioural interventions reviewed include aversive treatments and DRO scheduling, which are based on the appropriate application of positive and negative reinforcements. The work of Maier et al (1987) on today–tomorrow behavioural programming has been highlighted and the application of self-soothing skills discussed. The well-tried and tested stress-reducing strategies and anger control management techniques have been outlined, and social skills training have been emphasised both here and in the cognitive–behavioural techniques of Novaco's (1975) stress inoculation programme. Finally, a case has been made for raising the profile of future research and debate on theory and practice in relation to crisis intervention.

In the next chapter we will consider the controlling measures and management of violence and aggression from the practical perspective of policy formulation and production of guidelines to support staff in face-to-face confrontations. The provision of these frameworks is based on legal, moral and clinical requirements and is of major importance in establishing confidence in staff and offering a support framework in the event of litigation at a later stage.

7

Controlling measures and management

KEY POINTS

1. Policy formulation is central to the management of violence and aggression.
2. The management of violence and aggression is placed in the context of health provision and the notion of needs assessment.
3. Assessing needs at the point of crisis involves a number of factors.
4. Issues of control need to be addressed.
5. Countertransference can be problematic in the management of violence and aggression.

INTRODUCTION

Thus far, we have been concerned with attempting interventions that are aimed at defusing an aggressive situation by employing a number of techniques. In many of these circumstances, actual violence will be avoided and the aggression will dissipate without there being an incident. Many of these 'successes' become part of the health carer's everyday activity and are likely to go unrecorded (see Chapter 14). However, in some instances such diversionary tactics are not effective and the situation deteriorates further towards impending violence. It may be that as diversionary interventions are being attempted, the feedback received is negative and the person concerned begins to come to the conclusion that an outbreak of violence is increasingly more likely. Although attempts to defuse should continue, the decision maker ought to be thinking of contingency interventions at this stage, and assessing the situation in relation to the potential move to phase 3.

The main assumption of this chapter is that verbal interventions have been unsuccessful, there is an increasing probability of violence occurring, and therefore other alternatives should be considered. At this end point of phase 2, either the patient is about to erupt into violence or staff are going to attempt to take more physical control of the aggressor. In either event, this is a serious development; once physical control is attempted it must be safely achieved for all concerned.

This chapter, then, will deal with the issues involved in the decision to move from phase 2 to phase 3, in which physical action is required. The first major issue concerns policy formulation, from both national and organisational levels, as well as that based on personal codes of conduct. Policies should inform practice and staff should be aware of their organisation's guidelines in order to avoid transgressing them. Secondly, the assessment of need is vital at this point in time to ensure that the move to a physical intervention can be managed safely and the objectives achieved. This assessment will involve establishing the patient's current physical and mental health states as well as the extent of available resources, including staff and equipment. Thirdly, the issues involved in countertransference will be briefly outlined as these can influence the reinforcement of aggression and cause therapists to affect treatment outcomes adversely.

POLICY FORMULATION

Operationalising the management of violence and aggression to control individuals in the throes of attack requires skill and expertise. However, the skill and expertise must be grounded in an understanding and appreciation of policy.

National policies

First, one should refer to national policies that are directly concerned with the management of violence and aggression. These include publications such as those from the Royal College of Nursing (1972) offering practical advice, and publications that are only indirectly related, such as the Health and Safety at Work Act (Her Majesty's Stationery Office 1974), which states the law concerned with safe working conditions as well as practice. The Code of Practice (Her Majesty's Stationery Office 1993) is also a worthwhile national policy source. Although not statute law, such a document will be upheld in various courts, tribunals and enquiries as the benchmark of the profession's appropriate standards of care. We could also include here the UKCC (1996) Code of Conduct, which loosely sets out principles of professional practice, and can be both informative and important as a reference when devising policies on the management of violence and aggression.

Furthermore, operating within the guidelines given by these policies and codes is generally considered to equate with 'good practice'. Finally, although there is no one single law pertaining to the management of violence and aggression, from a professional health worker's point of view, a number of key legal principles have been set down, such as the use of minimum force (p. 146) and the least restrictive environment (p. 147), which should provide a basis. The importance of mentioning them here is that staff ought to know of these influences as they should govern one's practice in the face-to-face confrontation and, although they cannot be so specific as to guide every situation in every context, they can influence both organisational and individual policy development.

Organisational policy

There is a duty for an organisation to provide a policy on the management of violence and aggression, and although this duty may not be a legal requirement, it would certainly appear to us to be a moral obligation. The reasons for its importance are both complex and subtle, as there are implicit messages transmitted by the production, or non-production, of such a policy. If a policy is produced then an organisation is communicating to its staff that it recognises violence and aggression as a problem, that it faces up to this challenge, and that it recognises that the staff require guidance and that they will need support when they operate within the framework of the policy. Failure to produce a policy, on the other hand, sends out messages of a negative kind: that the organisation does not realise that violence and aggression are problems, or considers that they are merely 'part of the job', or that it is the responsibility of individuals as to how they respond, and in the event of things going wrong, that the organisation bears no liability. Furthermore, the production of a policy that is constructed in positive terms (i.e. what staff members *should do*), and explains what the management response will be, will encourage the development of preventive strategies. In the absence of a policy, there is a tendency during postincident reviews to emphasise what the staff member *should not have done,* which often, unless very skilfully managed, merely produces resentment.

Every organisation will have different policies for the management of violence and aggression depending upon their function, philosophy, objectives and responsibilities; therefore no attempt to be prescriptive will be undertaken here. However, there are some common themes that will be relevant to most organisations and these are outlined in Box 7.1.

Box 7.1 Common themes of policy development (adapted from Braithwaite 1992)

Common themes	*Rationales*
Violence is unacceptable	Irrespective of the organisation, violence will not be tolerated. This includes physical, verbal, or threatened violence.
Organisational response	This may include taking legal action against perpetrators, providing staff support systems, and developing preventive strategies.
Education and training	Training courses should be available for staff working in health care settings in which violence occurs, creating a culture of openness and learning.
Monitoring and recording	Organisations should have effective systems of recording acts of violence and aggression and should respond to patterns and trends in increasingly dangerous areas of work.
Resources	It should be recognised that there may be resource implications for the management of violence and aggression. Sometimes more effective management of existing resources can improve situations.

Staff involvement

In formulating organisational policy, it is wise to involve as many staff as possible, at least in gathering views about draft documents, as this will give staff a feeling of investment in making the policy work in practice. Furthermore, there should be a strong emphasis on joint working within both policy design and practice development – that is, acknowledging that staff in all disciplines are responsible, not only for preventing aggression, but also for assisting those who are attempting to control violent encounters. Collaborative work is also necessary between managers and clinicians, and organisational policy should make clear statements about joint responsibility.

Individual policy

We would like to finish this section with some brief statements on personal, or individual policy formulation for the management of violence and aggression. Everyone who faces violent encounters in their workplace has a valid point of view with regards to their own reactions and responses to such situations; however, we must also make an assumption that all staff have a desire to operate in a professional manner without recourse to retribution or vindictiveness. Given that, there follows that some central strands and rationales relating to personal policy can be identified; these are set out in Box 7.2.

Working in tandem, the organisational policy and the individual policy can function as part of the joint accountability mentioned above, in which

Box 7.2 Reflections in formulating personal policies

Personal reflections	*Rationales*
Knowledge required	It is important to know the organisation's policy on the management of violence and aggression as well as the Code of Practice and other professional guidelines. It is the individual's responsibility to keep abreast of publications and recent research relating to violence.
Safety parameters	Staff should know the parameters of safe practice and operate within them. This should also include operating so as to safeguard self, colleagues, patients, others, as well as the aggressor.
Limitations	Staff should know their own strengths and weaknesses as well as those of others involved in the encounter wherever possible. They should not make value judgements about these weaknesses.
Reflection	There is a need to be aware of fears and anxieties as well as to be able to critically appraise one's own performance. There is a need to understand countertransference issues.

both parties play a part in the overall prevention and management of violence and aggression.

NEEDS ASSESSMENT

At the moment when a situation is perceived as threatening, and whilst the person is applying defusing and diverting interventions, information is constantly being received about the unfolding scenario. This information is processed by those involved and decisions made are based on this synthesis. As the situation is perceived to be moving to a physical encounter, there are many factors that should be considered in the final decision. Many of these are dealt with in Chapters 8–11 on specific interventions. However, it is worth considering here, a number of issues that should be borne in mind and that, overall, can be said to contribute towards an assessment of need at the point of crisis.

Establishing baseline behaviour

As mentioned above, the information that has been received whilst approaching the situation, or during a verbal intervention aimed at de-escalating the situation, will already have informed the judgement of the decision maker. However, an attempt should also be made to establish a baseline of the situational encounter from both the patient's and staff members' perspectives. This may involve an assessment of behaviour, non-verbal cues and the verbal context.

Behavioural assessment

Although assessment of the encounter will be based on the evaluations undertaken during the preceding defusion attempts, these can be developed further by a quick assessment of behaviours that become apparent to the appraiser. For example, anger and hostility may be evident and you, as the health worker, should evaluate the level at which these are manifested. This assessment will be based on a subjective evaluation, rather than any attempt at objective scaling and it is worth noting the extent to which *you* feel that these are evident. Ask yourself questions such as: 'to what extent is the aggressor attempting to hold on to his anger, does he have some degree of control of it', or 'to what extent is the anger controlling him, and what dangers are presenting themselves'?

Non-verbal cues

Secondly, it is important to establish the baseline for non-verbal cues such as the proximity of the patient or how he encroaches into others' personal space. Check his posture and identify the degree of threat. To what extent does his facial expression indicate that he is about to become violent, is he clenching his teeth, and are there any facial grimaces or tics apparent? Also establish whether he undertakes eye contact and, if so, is it appropriate or is he staring menacingly? Does he make physical contact by jabbing a finger, or pushing someone, and does he make gestures of a threatening nature? Finally, ask yourself whether he is presenting any idiosyncratic behaviour that usually precedes violence, in this individual.

Verbal content

Thirdly, establish the baseline of verbal content: does he swear frequently, and if so, how often? What is his tone of voice like, the pitch, and the loudness? Does he repeat himself often, if so how frequently, and is he rational in his speech? To what extent is his verbal content depersonalised to include all staff as one entity (i.e. 'you lot') or himself as 'we'? Is he coherent?

By establishing a quick baseline of these behaviours you are then also in a position to identify any improvements or deteriorations in future evaluations. Once an intervention, particularly of a physical kind, is undertaken, it has to be seen through to an ultimate conclusion that will involve an assessment of whether he becomes calmer and more self-controlled. At this point, the baseline will be vitally important in gauging the accuracy of any change. There are no great claims made here about the scientific validity of such baseline observations; however, if subjectively noted for future reference they will aid prediction to some degree.

Identifying attitudes

Definitions of 'attitude'

Early usage of the term 'attitude' referred to a person's posture or the manner of his body stance in relation to a particular situation. However, it is more common these days for the term 'attitude' to be used with reference to a person's internal psychological state rather than this physical orientation (Warren & Jahoda 1973). Furthermore, in common usage, we are generally clear about our understanding of someone's 'attitude' used in this sense, and would have little difficulty in expressing what our attitude was to, say, our boss or a politician. Therefore, we may use both these semantic definitions of attitude, and incorporate them in both scientific and lay terms.

The relationship of attitude and behaviour

Much work has been undertaken to establish the relationship between a person's attitude and the extent to which it can influence behaviour. For example, if a person harbours a negative attitude towards someone, is he also more likely to behave negatively to them – maybe even subconsciously? The reader will probably have arrived at an answer that reflects the state of scientific research in this area, which basically concludes that, although a causal relationship between the two is difficult to establish empirically, the relationship is generally believed to exist (Wicker 1969). What this means is that, although we may have difficulty identifying the nature of the relationship, in everyday life, we assume that attitudes affect behaviour to some degree or another.

However, research has continued to uncover some major issues pertaining to this relationship; for example, there have been measurements taken of consistency between a given attitude and action directed at a particular target. Current thought suggests that there is a good deal of plasticity in people's attitudes, depending upon how questions relating to those attitudes are structured. Plous (1993, p. 63) noted: 'in many cases, the wording of a question significantly influences the answers people give. Consequently, it is worth paying close attention to the structure and context of questions'. This is of major importance to us in the management of violence and aggression; posing the right question to an aggressor, using the right structure, can elicit a change in the attitude that may underlie the aggressive behaviour. Thus, in examining violent encounters, one should attempt to establish the attitudes of all those involved, including staff, patients and others, as the individuals may be engaged in a self-reinforcing circuit of 'winding each other up' (Braithwaite 1992).

Making sense of violence

Some forms of violence are commonly said to be senseless or mindless, which gives the impression that some other types of violence may well be considered sensible or mindful. Formalised violence in the form of war, or justifiable violence as a self-defence strategy, may well fall into this latter category. However, much of the violence that we meet in health care settings appears to be of the first category: uncalled for, unjustified and irrational. We have already discussed (p. 27) approaching violent encounters with a view to attempting to understand the reasoning processes, or causative factors of such violence; here, we wish merely to highlight the importance of attempting to make sense of the encounter to provide information for the needs assessment.

Chapters 1–3 of this book have clearly indicated the wide and diverse theories relating to the causative factors, and roles and functions, of violence and aggression, and it is fair to say that there are as many causes of violence as there are outbursts. Aggression in health care settings may occur because of breakdowns in the social relations within that situation, for example, arguments occurring between family members waiting in a reception area; or it may be territorial or possessive in origin, in that particular chairs or spaces have been threatened or invaded. Aggression may be caused through altered mental states from psychiatric illnesses, drug-induced disinhibition, or substance abuse. To reiterate, the causes are numerous. What is important for the purposes of decision-making in dealing with the encounter is to attempt to bring a rational analysis to an otherwise apparently irrational act. Therefore, staff should evaluate the situation in relation to the pay-offs for the aggressor. Establish what the aggressor is getting out of this violent action; what are the rewards, who is supplying them and how can they be removed? Attempt to identify primary and secondary gains for the aggressor and, in the crisis phase, at least note them for future reference. Even grossly disturbed psychotics do not engage in violence for no reason – it is merely that we often have difficulty knowing what *their* reasons are.

Agreeable safety

Safety at work takes many forms, from the legal provision of the Health and Safety at Work Act (Her Majesty's Stationery Office 1974), which states 'it should be the duty of every employer to ensure, so far as is reasonably practicable, the health and safety and welfare at work of all his employees' (section two), to the development of safe working practices based on individual organisation policy formulation. However, we can clearly see a tension arising between what an organisation may consider to be a risk to safety and what an individual may perceive as such, when faced with a violent person. It is easy (as we often repeat) to make judgements regarding safety after the incident is concluded, or from a removed distance when one is not directly involved in the confrontation. Agreeable safety is concerned with the needs assessment by those who are involved at the point of crisis and who are embroiled within the encounter. It may well be that managers consider that they have a greater overall view of a situation but this does not bear in mind the individual involvement on a face-to-face basis for those immersed on the ground. An analogy can be drawn here to the exasperated football manager (and fans) observing from the grandstand but unable to influence the players on the pitch. What fun we can all have after the game is over, saying what we believe such and such a player *ought* to have done!

The objective in management is to establish an effective team, inclusive of all those on the periphery, that can function according to a planned strategy. The preparation for this will include all the items we have already referred to (training, provision of resources, etc.) and the ultimate boost will always be the support that the team are given. Finally, we must all realise that the decisions taken about face-to-face confrontation need to be firmly rooted in those who are there at that point in time. However, agreeable safety is a two-way notion; it does not exonerate individuals from all accountability, but insists that those individuals operate within the overall rules of engagement and work towards the most effective result for all concerned. Outlining the organisational approach to managing violence and aggression, Greaves (1994) has drawn together the multifaceted aspects of achieving safety; these include legal considerations as well as more practical approaches such as risk assessment. What is clear from this, is that, from a human perspective, when a physical intervention is about to be undertaken, the safety of all concerned lies at the heart of practice.

Documentation of incidents

As well as the clear physical safety issues, the importance of documentation cannot be overstated. Always ensure that records of incidents are completed in sufficient detail and that they:

1. are concise and meaningful
2. include the relevant care and management issues
3. include an explanation of the unfolding events
4. are based on significant observations, events and interpretations
5. include the reasons for the interventions
6. are factual
7. include references for evidence-based practice.

Raising confidence levels

Confidence is often thought of as self-assuredness, or self-reliance; however, although these are fair descriptions of what confidence is, in the context of social science, the semantic also involves a degree of trust. In fact, it is more accurately defined here as a belief in trustworthiness. To say that we have confidence in someone is to make a statement regarding how much we trust them to act in a certain manner or to show certain behaviours. Similarly, to have self-confidence means that we trust ourselves to act in a certain way or behave according to set rules. However, the concept of confidence involves a further dimension, which is basically concerned with balance. Although confidence is difficult to measure as it is a subjective evaluation that varies between individuals, over time and across contexts, it is a well-understood phenomenon on a person-to-person basis. We are all aware of when we are confident or not; although such confidence or lack of it may well be ill founded, we are all aware of the actual state. Furthermore, we can all recognise when we have confidence in others, or not, as the case may be. The balance of confidence also involves having too much or too little of it, either in relation to oneself, in others, or in the event. Again, we tend to be aware when we are underconfident, but unfortunately, tend to be unaware when we are overconfident.

What we wish to mention briefly here is the issue of raising confidence levels in oneself and others, and the role of this in approaches to the control and management of violence and aggression. The three main ingredients to raising confidence are training, support and experience.

Training

There are a number of studies that have clearly demonstrated a rise in clinician confidence following completion of recognised training courses for managing violence (for example, Rice et al 1989). This rise in confidence includes staff members' ability not only to manage violence effectively but also to prevent it, and reduce injuries and levels of assault. However, questions are raised regarding whether staff actually learn, remember and implement skills from these courses, or whether it is merely the gain in experience that produces these results.

Support

The provision of support frameworks also raises confidence. Frameworks can include alarm systems, staff support crisis teams, and postincident support from management services including counselling. What is important here, is the notion of safety in numbers; it is not specifically related to numbers of staff at a particular incident, but rather to an organisational response to violence and aggression.

Experience

Finally, experience of successful and unsuccessful interventions contributes towards raising confidence, either in a successful outcome, or in choosing a different approach to one that has failed. (Experience is dealt with more fully in Chapter 14.)

Communication

Concept and form of communication

The concept of communication is derived from a community; a community requires certain information, and the means by which this information is received and transmitted are clearly diverse. Different cultures have developed many different systems of transmitting this information, from the American Indian smoke signals to the modern-day fax. Contemporary communication systems include the traditional written message on paper (hard copy) but the world is also now awash with electronic computer e-mail (soft copy). The difference between the two, the hard and soft versions, illustrates very clearly the problem faced with all types of communication strategies: the problem of *meaning*.

Interpretation of meaning

Establishing the meaning of a piece of information that is communicated relies upon interpretation. However, we can all make the wrong interpretation, even from the right information. The problem of interpretation is further compounded by the context in which the message is relayed. For example, a request to go for a CAT scan may well send someone to a pet shop for some type of feline monitor but may also send others to a hospital radiography department for computerised axial tomography! Communications can go terribly wrong when there is a reliance on soft versions only, whether verbal and non-verbal forms. For instance, verbal messages can be misquoted, as in the children's game of Chinese whispers where a message such as 'send reinforcements, we are going to advance' may become 'send three and fourpence, we are going to a dance'! This is why verbal requests are usually preferred in the written (hard version) form. Non-verbal communication is far more easily misinterpreted and there are few amongst us who have not fallen foul of this. A wink of an eye may well be a prelude for sexual advancement – but take care, it may well be just a nervous tic!

Verbal and non-verbal strategies

Communication at the point of crisis in the management of violence and aggression will tend to be reliant upon both verbal and non-verbal messages. The information must be transmitted between all parties involved in the incident; therefore, one needs to be clear and concise in any verbal request and ensure that any non-verbal signs are well understood by all members. For example, a hand signal needs to be known and understood by all concerned. Remember, just as the aggressor is sending signals out regarding his state of mind, staff will also be communicating how they are feeling, and thus we have a rich source of information that can be misperceived by all those involved.

Consistency of action

All societies have rules and regulations that define acceptable behaviour and set limits to circumscribe what that society accepts as appropriate behaviour. Beyond this, action will be taken to control transgressors of those limits. This action, whatever it may be, must be consistent in order to be effective. In relation to action regarding the control and management of violence and aggression, the interventions applied must also be constant, in that they should be even-handed in their application. They should be fair and firm, but not excessive. They should marry up to the particular situation being faced. When organisations develop policies, they are done so in response to the setting of limits and there should be a consistent application of interventions across the organisation so that all those involved are aware both of these limits, and also of the agreed response when they are transgressed. If organisations do not respond consistently then boundaries become obscured and new precedents are set.

Consistency should also be aimed for, both between individuals and by individuals. If there is a recognised response to a given situation, this will become the established procedure, and known as such. Similarly, consistency by an individual will become a recognised and respected quality, as long as it is congruous and logical. The advantages of consistency include the knowledge that staff will be aware of the likely sequence of events in an unfolding situation, and thus will have a clearer idea of their role within it. However, one must caution against rigidity of action, which is counterproductive to the effective management of violence.

Anticipation

We have already discussed the function of adrenaline in preparing someone for action in response to a threatening situation (Chapter 1), noting that it raises the state of awareness and creates an expectancy within the person. When moving from a verbal intervention to a physical one, this physiological process naturally results in a state of anticipation prior to the action. Such anticipation can produce apprehension in staff, which may cause problems if not guarded against. If such expectancy becomes too negative, then outward manifestations become apparent that will be communicated to others, including the aggressor; this then becomes an additional problem that needs to be taken into consideration. Apprehension can be alleviated by engaging staff in a controlled action, for example, by asking them to do something or to make specific observations. Getting them to do something breaks the mental rumination that accompanies the apprehension of anticipation. Another approach is to talk quietly to the staff, using their names, to ensure that they are listening; this again creates a distraction from their own thoughts.

Moving from a verbal intervention to a physical one will usually involve moving from a state of inaction to action, and if there is an intervening period in which tensions have increased there can be an overreaction in the physical encounter. The combination of adrenaline ensuring that the body is in a state of preparation, and the mind being somewhat anxious, can result in someone using too much physical force. Therefore, great care is needed to reduce excessive anticipation and maintain self-control by staff members. This can be achieved by the use of calming and focusing methods with those involved and ensuring that anticipation remains a positive element rather than a negative one.

COUNTERTRANSFERENCE

Transference and countertransference

Transference is concerned with the feelings of the patient being projected on to the therapist; they may be positive emotions such as warmth and affection or may be negative ones such as hatred. Countertransference refers to the emotional reactions that the clinician has towards the patient; again these can be both positive or negative. The transference feelings of the patient may be derived from his illness, but equally may be caused by a personality clash, or even possibly by the interpersonal style of the therapist. Feelings expressed by the patient towards the clinician can then create the countertransference emotions in the therapist, which may exacerbate the situation. If a person becomes aggressive towards a health care worker, it is easy to see how that victim may then dislike the attacker; this may in turn cause the aggressor to reinforce his wish to assault. Thus, very quickly, issues of transference and countertransference can become locked into a self-reinforcing circuit of negativity. When dealing with violent and aggressive persons who become combatant, staff may also begin to adopt avoidance strategies and withdraw from interpersonal contact. This again can cause the patient to feel isolated and marginalised and creates a social distancing (Maier et al 1987) that further compounds the problem and fails to provide a situation conducive to therapeutic intervention.

Types of reaction

Denial

Countertransference issues *must* be addressed as they can negatively influence the assessment and evaluation of a patient, and therefore, affect the treatment strategy. Lion & Pasternak (1973) report a remarkable, and unusual, case where a therapist faced an armed patient who shot at him, but the gun misfired. Following a brief struggle, the patient desisted and began to cry. The therapist gave the gun to his secretary and escorted the patient through the grounds to the emergency admission unit. The therapist left the patient sitting alone in a room and asked the clerk to call for the duty psychiatrist. No information regarding the events was relayed to the psychiatrist or the clerk, and 2 hours later the duty psychiatrist found the patient alone in the room. The therapist explained his action by saying 'I did not want to influence your decision regarding the need to admit the patient' (Lion & Pasternak 1973, p. 130). As these authors noted: 'the denial can well be understood in the face of the crisis but is nonetheless glaring' (p. 130).

Overreaction

Denial is one reaction, but others can be just as problematic. Overreaction is another emotional countertransference response that can lead to clinicians overprescribing medication, setting too-severe limits, establishing unrealistic boundaries and defining unachievable objectives. These can then adversely affect the treatment outcomes.

Identification

Denial is a common response to anxiety-provoking situations; however, another is identification, in which staff may take a special interest in the patient. This may involve the staff member claiming that the aggressor is an 'interesting case' and will go out of his way for the patient, possibly buying small gifts or doing special favours for him, and listening to him recanting stories of past aggressive encounters without challenging the underlying conflicts. Identification can take many forms and vigilance is needed for staff working with aggressive clients.

Conflict revival

Another problematic countertransference issue concerns the revival of conflicts and tensions in the therapist's past. If a previous conflict is unresolved, then contemporary countertransference feelings can awaken the emotional turmoil causing distortions in judgements about the current patient. It is often the case that the therapist cannot access the relationship between these emotional responses and will require assistance in the form of counselling or supervision to resolve the conflict.

Dealing with countertransference

Countertransference problems are a particularly difficult area of work, and usually require senior staff, clinicians, supervisors or consultants to pursue them. One method of doing this was undertaken by Maier et al (1988; p. 10) who organised 'one hour sessions called Me-times, which were held at the am-pm change of shift, and are chaired by the unit chief, they are used to identify and resolve countertransference issues among all unit staff'. These sessions are used to identify such feelings as helplessness, anger, fear, rage and desires to punish. They are explored through opening statements such as 'what if ...', 'how do you feel about ...', and 'what I would do is ...' (Maier et al 1987). When these emotions are identified, it is absolutely crucial that they are not denigrated, dismissed or derided, and the senior staff must legitimate them as normal and understandable. Staff members must be made aware that it is safe to share these feelings and that they will not be sanctioned against in any way. Raising these issues and sharing these feelings will create a healthier therapeutic environment in which the staff and patient may begin to act with a positive regard.

CONCLUSIONS

Throughout phase 2 we have made many attempts to defuse and distract the patient from acting violently. These interventions have included, in Chapter 6, diversionary approaches and behavioural-type strategies. In this chapter, we have outlined management issues and have emphasised the necessity of policy formulation, which should draw on legal and professional codes of conduct, and we have made a claim for individual staff members to develop their own professional policy through learning and experience. We then set out what we believe are the main issues pertaining to a needs assessment of the management of violence and aggression; these include establishing a baseline of behaviours, identifying attitudes, making sense of irrational behaviour, establishing agreeable safety, raising confidence, communicative strategies, the role of consistency, and problems of anticipation. Finally, we have dealt with countertransference issues and the way in which they may be resolved.

We now conclude phase 2 in which verbal interventions have been attempted, and in more cases than not, they will have been successful. However, we must now deal with those situations in which defusion has failed and the aggressor begins the phase of attack, phase 3, in which more physical interventions are necessary.

PHASE 3

Phase of attack

8

Isolation techniques

KEY POINTS

1. Isolating patients who become violent is a commonly used technique.
2. The methods of isolating patients are variations on the theme of seclusion.
3. There are seven phases to the appropriate use of seclusion.
4. Isolating patients who destroy property can be an emergency control measure.
5. There are advantages and disadvantages to the use of isolation techniques.

INTRODUCTION

In the last chapter we saw how a violent situation may deteriorate and idenfitified some strategies to contain it. If an actual attack becomes more likely in a situation, then the necessity for some type of physical restraint is deemed to be more probable. This may well take the form of the formally approved C&R technique (see Chapter 9) or be more organisationally driven and informal. Once physical control has been established, however, in some cases, the person continues to struggle or is deemed a persisting threat to the safety of others, and needs to be isolated from those he could harm. (Although in this book we depict physical restraint as following isolation techniques, in some cases they occur in the reverse order as we will see.)

The debate about whether to isolate patients who become violent or aggressive by using seclusion revolves around those authors who perceive its use to be a therapeutic intervention, those who consider it to be a form of punitive sanction, and those who believe it to be merely a method of containment in the absence of alternatives. Some establishments have ceased to use it altogether and have developed non-seclusion policies, whilst others have suggested that the alternatives are equally, or more, unacceptable. However, we do not wish to engage in an academic debate on the philosophical constructs of the use of seclusion in this chapter. Instead, we wish merely to acknowledge that in the throes of combat, some individuals and organisations accept that the use of seclusion and other forms of isolation are acceptable for the prevention of serious harm to others. The interested reader who wishes to review the literature on seclusion more fully is referred to the works by Alty & Mason (1994), Angold (1989), Fisher (1994), Hodgkinson (1985), and Mason (1995).

In this chapter, we wish to focus on the various methods of isolationary situations that can occur in many types of mental health setting. Some of these are accepted professional techniques whilst others are practices that have developed in response to organisational requirements. The different types of seclusionary practices will be set out and the specific issues relating to the use of seclusion will be discussed in relation to the problems that can occur. This discussion will place isolation in the context of the issue relating to the least restrictive measure. A plan of action will be described in order to forestall the development of problems; although policies on seclusion differ from establishment to establishment, there are central themes that emerge and overlap across contexts. In phase 3, during which assault is under way, there is an urgent need to establish emergency control and although physically holding (see Ch. 9) may already have been achieved, for the purpose of establishing seclusion, there are practical steps that have to be taken for safe control and transportation to the seclusion room. Therefore, we will present some practical pointers for getting the occupant into the seclusion room safely and getting the staff out of the room unscathed. Finally, there are both advantages and disadvantages to isolating patients and these will also be outlined.

METHODS OF ISOLATIONARY PRACTICE

Persons who become violent and aggressive may need to be isolated in order to protect others from harm. If someone is in the throes of attacking another person, then ensuring he is safely isolated away from those he seeks to injure is of paramount importance. However, some have argued that isolation can be used in both phases 2 and 3, during which time either the patient is deteriorating or he has become assaultive. There are a number of ways in which a disturbed violent patient can be isolated.

The quiet room

The quiet room is, by and large, indistinguishable from a seclusion room except for the use of 'softer' terminology and differences in design that would be expected in differing settings. Joshi, Capozzoli & Coyle (1988) described a quiet room in these terms: 'they are equipped with audio-visual monitoring systems ... ensuring constant visual contact and verbal interaction ... the door possesses a non-breakable viewing window ... rooms are devoid of any furniture or equipment ...' (pp. 642–3). Hickerson & Garrison (1991), in describing quiet room utilization patterns, merely put the word 'seclusion' in brackets following the term 'quiet room' thus clearly indicating that they were interchangeable.

The quiet room is used for the following reasons:

1. as part of a graded continuum to reduce sensory stimuli
2. to divert aggressive behaviour
3. to encourage patients' internal control
4. as a method of disrupting provocation.

The programme here must be seen as therapeutic and it is advised that patients and relatives should be given the opportunity to discuss the use of the quiet room, and make a visit to it, on admission.

Room restriction

Between the use of seclusion and time-out as a behaviour modification technique (see below) lies the idea of room restriction. This is a preplanned routine that involves informing the patient in advance of his unacceptable behaviour that will lead to room restriction. However, unlike time-out, it is not used necessarily to extinguish undesirable behaviour but also to allow the person to work through his emotions and develop alternative ways of coping (Gentilin 1987). Room restriction, unlike seclusion, is never used impulsively without an assessment and a preplanned phase in which the patient is informed as to when it is likely to be used. Therefore, it is neither time-out nor seclusion.

Room restriction is usually used for the following reasons:

1. when patients need an external control over their behaviour
2. when patients need boundaries to be set
3. when patients are testing the institutional system
4. when patients need feedback of their behaviour
5. when patients need clear and consistent messages about the role of others.

We can see that within the room restriction rationale, there is a developmental ethos in which the patient learns to deal with his emotions and a period of personal growth is anticipated. A room restriction care plan could be as shown in Box 8.1.

Box 8.1 Room restriction plan (adapted from Gentilin 1987)

Name	*Date*
Reason for RR	Verbal aggression towards others
Interventions	Periods with staff on one-to-one, 45 minutes, twice per shift. Patient to keep diary of feelings whilst on RR. Newspapers and books to be given as behaviour improves
Association	Periods of time out of room in association with other members of staff and ward community
Physical care	Washing, bathing and exercise – two periods per day. Toileting as requested
Objectives	The patient to understand his emotions more fully and the impact his behaviour may have on others
Evaluation	The RR programme will be evaluated during each shift. Date and time to be recorded
Termination	The patient will complete the RR programme and if evaluation indicates, the RR will be terminated

RR = room restriction.

Limit setting

Limit setting is another isolationary manoeuvre that can restrict the movement of the aggressive patient. In its widest sense it can be all-inclusive and incorporate every aspect of psychiatry including 'mental hospitalization, seclusion, one-to-one observations, restraints and medication' (Gair 1980, p. 16). However, in its more restricted sense, it refers to the establishment of boundaries within which the patient is expected to operate. For it to function adequately, the authority to set limits is delegated to those in the emergency situations in which speed of intervention is paramount. It has several principles to guide its usage:

1. Nursing responsibility for limit setting is supported by the patient care team.

2. Nursing staff must be aware of this multidisciplinary support but must also operate in a professional manner.
3. Staff should receive some training in limit setting.
4. Limit setting calls for plausible conclusions.
5. Patients should be made aware of the boundaries in which they are expected to behave.

Time-out

Time-out as an isolation technique is probably the most abused term in mental health. Time-out is part of the behavioural science known as behaviour modification. It refers to the removal of a positive reinforcer that is rewarding the patient's unwanted behaviour. It has three central aspects that distinguish it from seclusion. First, time-out can involve the removal of a positive reinforcer for a specified period of time immediately following the presentation of the undesirable behaviour. In this use of time-out, it is the external positive reinforcer that is removed and not the patient. The second aspect is the partial removal of a patient from the source of the positive-reinforcing stimulus, but not out of its environment. The third element is the complete removal of the patient from the positively reinforcing environment. However, despite the very clear differences, the term 'time-out' is often used for convenience when someone wishes to lock a patient away without initiating the seclusion procedure with the accompanying paperwork that ensues. It can also be abused, as when time-out is used merely as a 'scientific term' in order to put on a front to dismiss negative responses from some quarters.

To safeguard against the misuse both of the term time-out and of patients themselves, three questions should be posed to any staff members claiming to be using it. Firstly, what is the reinforcing stimuli from which removal is planned? Secondly, what is the undesirable behaviour that it is being used to extinguish? Thirdly, what is the specified period of time-out as per the behaviour modification plan? The reason for this safeguard is that its use is against the spirit of the Code of Practice, so that staff using time-out inappropriately, are vulnerable to accusations of professional misconduct. There are many published works on time-out with a number discussing its relationship with seclusion. A later article by Landau & MacLeish (1988) brought the legal situation into sharp focus with its title 'When does time-out become seclusion, and what must be done when this line is crossed?' Although this refers to American state legislation, its principles are apposite for Britain.

A behavioural modification time-out plan would be followed by an evaluation of the subject, establishing any equipment that would be used, and mapping out precisely the procedure. In extinguishing, or suppressing the aggression in a young girl, the plan may follow the pattern shown in Box 8.2.

Box 8.2 Time-out plan for extinction/suppression of aggressive behaviour

1. Establish baseline. First eight sessions, nurses are taught to ignore non-injurious aggression
2. Reaffirm baseline. Ignore non-injurious aggression and reinstruct those nurses who fail
3. Intermittent 5 minute TO for assault on another for 25 sessions. Random time-sample obtained
4. Intermittent 15 minute TO for assault on another for 20 sessions. Observations made of sessions
5. Continuous 5 minute TO as above
6. Extinction procedure, ignore all but the most dangerous aggressive behaviour
7. Continuous 5 minute TO to repeat above phases
8. Extinction to repeat 6
9. Continue programme

TO = time-out.

The seclusion room

A seclusion room is a designated room on the unit; it should be purpose built. Gutheil & Daly (1980) argued for a non-clinical focus to the design of the room, by which they meant that it should be practical for the purpose it is intended. However, they were also aware of the close relationship between the room itself and the attitude adopted to patients whilst they were resident in the room. This non-clinical focus would begin with a concern about the strength of the patient, who in the frenzy of a psychotic breakdown, appears to be able to summon immense strength. There is also concern about access to weapons obtained from a disturbed patient destroying the fittings in a room; Gutheil and Daly argued for grills over lighting and windows as well as carefully constructed joins to prevent the patient from pulling such fittings apart. They concluded: 'the aim is to keep the occupant safe in the room and to maintain the room safe from the occupant ...' (Gutheil & Daly 1980, p. 270).

Throughout the psychiatrised world, the seclusion room is relatively standard with only minor modifications. It is typically 4–5 metres by 2–3 metres with little or no furnishings; it may have a mattress on the floor with strong bedding that is difficult to tear or it may have a moulded plastic bed fixed to the ground with ordinary blankets and sheets. Windows and lighting may have protective coverings and observation slits will be located in the doors and/or adjacent rooms. Modern seclusion rooms will have heat and ventilation controls outside the room and possibly toileting facilities as an annexe. Less contemporary designs usually have disposable urinals and bedpans within the room.

Patients are secluded against their wishes and the door is locked. A seclusion record must be maintained and there are a number of examples in the literature for those interested (Justic 1993; Kendrick & Wilber 1986;

Strawser 1994). Typically, they will be of a format such as that shown in Figures 8.1 and 8.2. The seclusion room, again typically, is used for only very short periods, in the extremes of violent behaviour, when all else has failed and there is a significant risk of harm to others. Once the patient has settled, he is immediately allowed out of the room.

Open-area seclusion

Open-area seclusion is a situation where a 'patient is placed in a segregated (and locked) area together with staff members, but the patient is never isolated alone in a single locked room for seclusion' (Bjorkly 1995; p. 148). The claim for this type of isolationary practice is that the time in open-area seclusion is used psychotherapeutically for teaching improved interpersonal communication and developing coping strategies. This is unlike seclusion in which destimulation is expected and the patient becomes calm and compliant. This psychotherapeutic approach is based on behaviourism, cognitive therapy and crisis intervention (Bjorkly 1995). There is a four-staged approach to this method of isolation:

1. The initial phase involves the patient being removed, voluntarily or by physical force, to the open area.
2. The second phase incorporates a calming-down period during which the person is psychologically assessed.
3. The third phase involves establishing the motives for the assaultive behaviour and learning from the experience.
4. The fourth phase establishes reintegration of the patient into the ward community.

There are five components to the psychotherapeutic use of open-area seclusion:

1. containment of the violent behaviour
2. destimulation
3. reality orientation
4. behavioural responsibility
5. solving problems with an emphasis on alternative action.

Intensive care areas

Another method of isolating violent persons is to designate an intensive care area (ICA), in which a small area of the ward is locked off from the remainder of the community. This then operates as a self-contained unit comprising of bedrooms, toilet and bathing facilities, as well as recreational and occupational areas. Up to four patients may be managed in these areas, usually with a staffing ratio of one to one. However, this all depends on the

Date	Day No.	Serial No.							

Unit	Patient's Name	Ward	Patient's number	Person ordering seclusion Name Signature

RMO: Primary nurse	Psychologist Social worker
Seclusion initiated: Date Time	Seclusion terminated: Date Time
Name, date and time informed to be entered below	

RMO: Date/Time	Registrar	Snr manager	Psychologist	Social Worker

Reason for seclusion Initiating/Continuing
Document any PRN medication given

Name of drug	Route		Time given			Name of nurse			Form 38	Form 39	Sec 62

RMO involved Yes/No	Clinical manager Yes/No	UGM Yes/No
Type of room	Type of bed	Type of bedding
Clothing worn	Personal possessions	Access to toilet
Related to incident no.	Complaints made Yes/No	Complaint No.

REVIEW PROCESS			
Immediate review/within first 4 hours: Comments	Personnel:	Name	Signature
	RMO/REG		
	Snr manager		
	Nurse		
	Social worker		
	Psychologist		
Same repeated for 4, 8, 12, 24 hour reviews			

	AM			PM			NIGHTS		
	Level of nurse			Level of nurse			Level of nurse		
	1st.	2nd.	N.A.	1st.	2nd.	N.A.	1st.	2nd.	N.A.
Female staff									
Male staff									
Nurse I/C signature and Grade									

Figure 8.1 Format for a seclusion record.

<table>
<tr><td colspan="2">Name:</td><td>Day No:</td><td colspan="2">Serial No:</td><td colspan="2">Date:</td></tr>
<tr><td rowspan="2">Time</td><td colspan="2" rowspan="2">Observation text at least every 15 minutes</td><td colspan="3">Cumulative times in/out of seclusion</td><td rowspan="2">Name/ signature</td></tr>
<tr><td colspan="2">IN</td><td>OUT</td></tr>
<tr><td>09:30</td><td colspan="2"></td><td colspan="2"></td><td></td><td></td></tr>
<tr><td></td><td colspan="2"></td><td colspan="2"></td><td></td><td></td></tr>
<tr><td></td><td colspan="2"></td><td colspan="2"></td><td></td><td></td></tr>
<tr><td></td><td colspan="2"></td><td colspan="2"></td><td></td><td></td></tr>
<tr><td colspan="7">Repeated through the 24-hour clock</td></tr>
<tr><td>Totals</td><td colspan="2"></td><td colspan="2"></td><td></td><td></td></tr>
<tr><td colspan="3" rowspan="8">Daily review 1 comments</td><td>Personnel</td><td colspan="2">Name</td><td>Signature</td></tr>
<tr><td>RMO/REG</td><td colspan="2"></td><td></td></tr>
<tr><td>Snr manager</td><td colspan="2"></td><td></td></tr>
<tr><td>Nurse</td><td colspan="2"></td><td></td></tr>
<tr><td>Social worker</td><td colspan="2"></td><td></td></tr>
<tr><td>Psychologist</td><td colspan="2"></td><td></td></tr>
<tr><td>UGM</td><td colspan="2"></td><td></td></tr>
<tr><td colspan="7">Repeated for each review</td></tr>
</table>

Figure 8.2 Observation chart for a seclusion record.

severity of the clinical conditions and the strengths and weaknesses of the staff. Craig, Ray & Hix (1989) argued for the least restrictive environment within a multivariate entity. This, they argued, could include a suite of secure rooms including a seclusion room, a restraint room, a bathroom and a central area linking the others together. The idea of this is that the patient could be managed in the least restrictive way within this suite of rooms by moving him from one to the other as the situation dictated.

Kinsella, Chaloner & Brosnan (1993) reported on an ICA within a medium secure unit; in this they claimed some success in managing violent and aggressive people in a two-bed unit with relatively high levels of individual freedom.

The rationale for using an ICA includes the following:

1. It provides an area in which violent patients can be isolated but not left alone.
2. Nurses can observe the patients at all times.
3. Nurses can respond quickly to patients' needs.
4. The ICA is a controlled environment.

An ICA schedule may be designed as in Box 8.3.

Box 8.3 Intensive care area schedule

Name	*Date*
Physical safety for patients	Check items that can be used for self-injury and suicide (matches, lighters, etc.)
Physical safety for staff	Control for access to weapons, both opportunistic and fashioned
Phychological interventions	Engage when appropriate. Observe for signs of deterioration. Divert attention where possible. Occupy in other activities
Observations	15 minute time-sample record. Baseline assessments followed up with periodic evaluations
Reintegration	Discuss behaviour required for reintegration into ward community. Establish external factors that affect reintegration (i.e. ward community). Avoid allowing the patient to become institutionalised
Daily activities	Ensure adequate food, liquid, washing, exercise and sleep

ISSUES INVOLVED IN ISOLATING PATIENTS

Aggressive patients who are attacking others, or who are destroying property, are engaging in out-of-control actions that are in themselves both disturbing and frightening. When others are being injured, there is an urgency to intervene to rescue the damaged party and to prevent further harm. Similarly, when windows are being smashed and furniture broken, there is a sense of necessity to stop the destruction although, clearly, property is more dispensable than people. In these situations, there are several issues that we need to be aware of and specific problem areas that arise in relation to isolationary practices.

Patient safety

The first issue refers to the safety of the aggressive patient. If the attack is on property, then the main concern is with the obvious access to weapons (i.e. glass, broken furniture) that could be used either to inflict self-harm or to attack others. When a frenzied attack subsides, there may be intense feelings of despair and despondency at the damage caused and the apparent hopelessness of the problem. In these moments, there can be a sudden attempt at suicide or self-injury using glass, knives or electrocution. If the aggressor has been isolated within the area that is being destroyed, then he is at risk during this period of being alone. Furthermore, the patient may harm himself quite by accident during these periods of destruction. For example, smashing light fittings appears to be a favourite activity and glass and shards of fittings can rain down and cause injury.

Therefore, one always needs to balance the safety of the patient against the possibility of leaving him to exhaust himself on property destruction. The damage caused to the patient may well take other forms during these phases of property destruction; for instance, there may be delayed consequences in the form of personal revenge by other patients who have had property damaged, or financial liability, as some organisations charge patients for the damage caused.

Staff safety

A second issue involves the safety of staff. Staff members intervening in a situation of property destruction may find themselves facing a very disturbed individual equipped with a weapon. Equally, they may be injured more by accident, slipping or tripping, as they avoid thrown items or flailing clubs and batons. Although working in mental health settings involves, from time to time, the outbreak of violence and aggression, there is a requirement under the Health and Safety at Work Act 1990 for the working environment to be a safe one. This requirement encompasses not only systems and policies to safeguard staff, but also the provision of training and education. In the arena of managing violence and aggression, the latter aspect is of vital importance; it may include formal training in such courses as C&R (see Chapter 9) or more informal ward-based training.

Therapeutic outcome

A third issue in isolation techniques concerns the best therapeutic outcome. There is always considerable debate as to whether one particular mode of isolation is more therapeutic than another and a degree of personal choice is usually noted. Whereas one line of argument may suggest that seclusion alone in a locked room provides the most destimulating environment, another claims that it is more therapeutic for nurses to remain in attendance. Some suggest that at the moment of psychiatric crisis, the patient should not be left isolated, whilst others report that nurses in constant attendance provide a too-intense and often provoking situation. The best therapeutic outcome is often not appreciated in the short term but requires a longer-term assessment.

Injures, deaths and medication in emergency situations

Some specific problems arise as a consequence of isolating patients. The first concerns injuries that may be sustained by patients who are being secluded. These injuries can result in official complaint and may be the subject of investigation and litigation. Struggling with violent patients is clearly a dangerous enterprise that can result in injuries sustained by overzealousness, overreaction through fear, and also quite by accident. Secondly, there have been a number of deaths of patients who have been isolated and, again, although some of these are quite natural, in other cases they appear to directly result from being isolated. Leaving patients locked in an area alone, with staff beyond sight and sound of the patient, can be a dangerous practice. Thirdly, the use of medication and isolation of patients is particularly problematic, as in emergency situations, disturbed and violent patients may receive pro re nata (PRN) medication at the time of being isolated. In these circumstances, patients are vulnerable and should have a nurse in visual contact during periods of sedation.

PHASES OF ISOLATION

In this section we wish to focus upon the controlled use of seclusion through a series of phases in which the staff are deciding on the sequence of events, rather than reacting to the patient. From the previous section, we note four principles that underscore actions in establishing the seclusion of a patient: (a) safety of the patient, (b) safety of staff, (c) best therapeutic outcome and (d) professional conduct. The phases are not clearly delineated by boundaries but overlap and fuse with each other, therefore the process of assessments within one phase can also be undertaken in others. Also, although we are here using the process of seclusion as a form of isolation as an example, the same guidelines could be used for establishing any of the isolation techniques mentioned above, with minor qualifications. These qualifications are, that all the points within each phase of the seclusion may not be relevant for each and every episode of an isolation procedure. They are thus offered as guidelines to be individualised according to specific situations.

There are seven phases to the seclusion procedure, namely planning, initiation, acclimatisation, intermediation, termination, reintegration and milieu intervention.

Planning phase

There is much that can be incorporated within this first phase. For example, training and education of staff at induction into the ward, as well as in-service training at follow-up, are important aspects of overall planning. However, here we wish to focus more specifically on the practical aspects at the clinical interface as a crisis develops.

Staff discussion

To begin with, a forum should be established for staff to discuss the whole aspect of the use of seclusion on their unit. This should encourage the debate of positive and negative feelings, as well as develop an open agenda regarding the procedure for secluding a patient. Specific behaviours and events likely to warrant seclusion and alternatives could be talked through as appropriate. These behaviours and events, which are often emergency, or serious situations that can evoke considerable anxiety and stress in staff, could be aired in these forums (Gentilin 1987). When a specific seclusion episode is about to occur, the planning phase should incorporate a discussion of the actual plan. The latter should be made clear to everyone involved in the procedure and an opportunity should be given for questions and reassurance. The patient should be identified and the reason for the seclusion stated. This should also include information on previous history of the patient, the likely anticipated behavioural response, the age, size and strength of the person, and the expected level of control that will be required. However, it is also important to omit unnecessary information and avoid emotive embellishments, which are likely only to increase the tension for all concerned (Kendrick & Wilber 1986).

Staff assignment

Staff members should be assigned to specific tasks, making an assessment of the nurse's strengths and weaknesses in relation to those of the patient. For example, if the patient has a special relationship with a particular member of staff, then this could be used if considered appropriate. Similarly, if a staff member is prone to become overstressed in such physical situations it would be wise to allocate him to another responsibility (e.g. drawing up medication or observing other members of the ward community).

Having assessed the strengths and weaknesses of both the staff and the patient, it is appropriate to continue with a brief assessment of opportunities and threats that may develop. For example, in their disturbed state, patients may well have partly undressed themselves, or have become isolated in a corner of a room, both of which could be considered as opportunities for intervention. However, a patient could also have some peer support from fellow patients which must be considered a threat.

If staff members are trained in C&R then this would be used. However, if not, then one member of staff should be assigned to each of the patient's limbs and a fifth member assigned as spokesperson and leader of the operation and also to control the patient's head. The spokesperson should be the person who verbally interacts with the patient at all times during the first two phases, should direct the movements of the team, observing for cues from both the staff and the patient, and should signal the exit from the seclusion room. In the planning phase, the spokesperson should be aware of this role and be given the opportunity to discuss it.

Checks and precautions

There should be a check for possible safety hazards on all staff involved; such items as pens, name tags, watches, necklaces, rings, glasses should be removed. Any non-removable rings should be taped over. A check of the seclusion room should be carried out for any items that should not be there and ensuring that any items that will be required are placed ready (e.g. bed clothes). Long hair should be tied back and loose items in pockets removed.

This planning phase should be carried out in the shortest possible time and away from the patient's view.

Initiation phase

The initiation phase will always be unique for each situation and therefore, require differing responses to match. However, having said that, there will be key elements that overlap and should be considered as the situation is being observed or approached.

Assessment

An assessment of the behavioural indicators should first be undertaken; this includes the extent of the violence being carried out, the possible harm to self or others, the property being destroyed, the access to weapons (e.g. glass) and the location of both the patient being secluded and others in the vicinity (Bjorkly 1995).

The approach assessment should also include an evaluation of the patient's mental condition as far as can be ascertained and judgements should be made about the most appropriate approach. It may be that a show of force in the form of a 'wall of personnel' may subdue the patient who can then be escorted to the seclusion room quietly (Gair 1980). Alternatively, it may be that more personnel will actually exacerbate the situation and the patient becomes more aggressive and resistant. One situation may call for the staff team members to meander closer to the patient from various directions and wait for the spokesperson to signal the 'take-down', whilst another situation may call for an urgent rush. It may be appropriate to request the patient to go into seclusion calmly, or this may merely provide the patient with a warning signal and cause more harm than good.

Approaching the patient

The objective at this stage is to adopt a calm, effective and firm approach and conduct the procedure in a professional manner. If time allows, the area should be cleared of all other patients and an extra staff member assigned to act as observer for the 'take-down' who can give feedback at a later stage about any difficulties encountered. If the patient is offered the opportunity to walk quietly to the seclusion room, then only a few seconds should be given to comply. When the agreed signal is given by the spokesperson, the staff secure their allocated limbs and gently move the patient backwards, lowering him to the floor. Minimum force should be applied to control the patient and there should be no attempt to insult, humiliate or cause further pain to the patient. When the patient is secured on the floor, then further staff may be summoned to move him to the seclusion room. It is wise, at this stage, to remove the patient's shoes to prevent any further injury through kicking.

Moving the patient

If a degree of compliance is noted, then the move to the room can be undertaken by staff members maintaining a hold on each arm with the patient walking. If this is not the case he may need to be carried. In any event, there should be no release of the limbs until the patient is in the seclusion room, irrespective of whether he says he will now comply if staff let go. Once in the seclusion room, the patient should be placed face down on the bed and, for safety, any of the following items removed: belts, shoes, tie, various pocket contents, etc. Whilst the patient is face down, with his head to one side, the legs are folded one across the other (cross-legged) with the top one held to secure the one beneath, the legs can now be secured by one staff member. It should be noted here that this position is usually quite comfortable for the majority of people but that severely overweight patients can have their breathing restricted in this position, and therefore, in these patients it should be avoided (Tardiff 1989). The patient should be observed at all times for difficulty with breathing or signs of collapse. At a prearranged signal, the head and arms are then released and the staff quickly exit the room. The final person holding the crossed legs should now release them and step sharply out of the room. A member of staff should have the key ready in the seclusion room door, which should be shut and locked. On release, the secluded patient who is held in this position is usually quite slow to get up, therefore, the last staff member has time to exit.

The issue and procedure for emergency medication at this stage is dealt with in Chapter 11. A staff member should stay in close observation of the patient to ascertain his reaction to the seclusion and to ensure that the patient's breathing is satisfactory. Any equipment needed should now be collected, such as a sphygmomanometer, drinking utensils and so on. These should not be in the seclusion room but readily accessible.

Acclimatisation phase

In the first few moments of the seclusion, the patient's emotions are likely to be running high. There may be banging on the door, shouting of abuse, screaming and tearing of clothes, or an attempt to destroy the room. However, the patient may also hide under the bed clothes and be emotionally upset. In this early phase, the patient is usually quite angry and feels humiliated, and visual contact (VC) should be maintained with or without the use of medication (Baradell 1985). The VC should be continued until the patient's mental state is calmer and his behaviour less disturbed.

This acclimatisation phase may last a few minutes or a couple of hours, and during this time it has been reported that some of the patient's signs and symptoms actually worsen whilst in seclusion (Mason 1995). In this period, there is little point in attempting to engage the patient in any therapeutic discourse; instead, any communication should be concrete and directive but also stated in a kind and considerate manner. The VC should be maintained until the patient's behaviour becomes calmer, although this is not an indication of the state of his internal feelings. An assessment is needed here to gauge the level of stimulation that is required to help the patient calm down. External noise should be reduced and activity outside of the seclusion room should be minimal.

Intermediation phase

In this phase, the patient's behaviour becomes manageable and work may begin on his internal feelings. The patient becomes highly attuned to the attitudes and behaviour of staff during this phase, and therefore, the staff are crucial in determining the likely duration of the seclusion. The patient also becomes very sensitive to sound and a further assessment is needed as to the level of stimulation that is required by the patient.

During this phase, it will almost certainly be necessary to re-enter the seclusion room, for any number of routine reasons. The patient should be informed to sit or lie on the mattress and remain there as the staff enter the room. Avoid hovering over the patient and adopt a sitting or squatting position, in this phase, to make eye contact on an equal level. Also avoid threatening body language such as folded arms, hands on hips and sudden movements. Equally, avoid suspicious posturing such as hands behind back and glancing furtively around. Offer reassurance to the patient and portray a quietly confident and professional manner. Withdraw from the room calmly whilst maintaining observation of the patient.

Early on in this phase, the patient needs to know the reason for the seclusion and to be informed that it was not performed for punitive reasons, but to help him regain internal control. Alternative behaviours may be discussed and coping strategies identified. The patient needs to know what is required for the termination of seclusion and when it is likely to happen in relation to his mental state. Inform the patient that frequent observations will be made and that it is expected that his behaviour will improve. Help him to cope with anxiety and the loss of personal freedom. Personal belongings can be allowed into the seclusion room at this stage if the patient's mental state warrants it, and reassurance should be offered about how others on the ward perceive him. As the patient improves, he can be set certain goals and take on more responsibility (Bjorkly 1995).

Termination phase

The assessment for terminating seclusion should be based on the patient's overall mental health state, his response to seclusion, and the insight gained about both the inappropriateness of the behaviour that led to seclusion and the development of alternative strategies. If the level of internal control is deemed to be sufficiently re-established, then an increase in independence can be offered. This should accompany more activities and further assessments. The actual decision to terminate a seclusion regimen should be a group decision involving the multidisciplinary team if possible, and if not, then involving two or more nurses on the unit.

Assessment

Assessing a patient's suitability for release from seclusion can involve any number of approaches that can be drawn from the wealth of literature on mental health assessments. However, a number of factors are extremely important when assessing a patient for termination of seclusion. These relate to the severity of the signs and symptoms whilst in seclusion. It has been noted that some patients actually deteriorate whilst in seclusion before they improve (Mason 1995) and great care must be taken to make accurate assessments on a regular basis. Patients may be verbally abusive and threatening whilst in seclusion and the risk of revenge attacks is all too great if seclusion is terminated too soon. If a patient is suspicious, labile in mood and provocative, then caution should be exercised and if he is allowed out of seclusion then intense observation should be maintained.

Reintegration phase

It may well be appropriate for seclusion to cease and the patient to be allowed directly back into the ward community without further consideration. However, a more gradual stepwise approach is usual. One-to-one supervision may be required while the patient is being assessed, or he may be allowed to take meals or coffee breaks with other patients as a preliminary step. The patient may well feel embarrassed or anxious regarding re-entry and reassurance will be required. The use of seclusion should be reinforced as a method of caring for the patient during a crisis that is now over and the fact that the patient has regained control should be rewarded (Chu & Ryan 1987). It will be necessary still to observe and assess the patient for signs of deterioration whilst out in the ward area and make interventions when necessary.

The explosive nature of violence and aggression is such that its predictability is extremely limited; it is often only in retrospect that signs and symptoms appear important. The patient's orientation to the ward should be monitored and his acceptance by peers closely observed. If the intensity of the ward relationships are overpowering then the patient can regress very rapidly, therefore, the expression of emotions is helpful in determining the patient's current mental state. Levels of agitation can rise quickly and there should be swift intervention to prevent any deterioration. However, there can also be a negative reaction to staff approaches, which should be dealt with sensitively and without confrontation.

Milieu intervention phase

It is important to evaluate the overall ward milieu in response to the patient re-entering the community. There may be open hostility towards the secluded patient and the possibility of revenge attacks if he had hurt someone in the initial violence, or he may be excluded from others and feel rejected. In either case, there is a need for intervention and further observation to protect the patient. On the other hand, ward members may feel threatened by the secluded patient, which will increase their stress and they will require reassurance. Community meetings may help, as would engaging the secluded patient in communal activities.

The ward dynamic is often intuitively 'felt' by those involved in the day-to-day community rather than empirically measured by some ward environment scale and experienced staff can often perceive that all is not as usual. Levels of arousal may be different, or there may be a higher degree of restlessness by staff and patients. Aggressive posturing may be observed and there may be furtive glances between patients, which indicates that something is amiss. In studies of ward environments, it is noted that the staff/patient dynamic is crucial in disrupting or stabilising a ward.

EMERGENCY ISOLATION CONTROL

In other contexts, it is the patient who dictates the sequence of events, at least initially, and the main thrust of the staff members' actions is geared towards regaining control of the situation. If a violent person is directing aggression towards property, perhaps smashing windows or ripping down fixtures and fittings, and no other person is directly at risk, then there may well be a case for a non-interventive approach in the first instance. In this scenario, the destructive person could be isolated by locking off access to other areas and exits from the area in which they are located.

Visual contact should be maintained wherever possible and support should be summoned. Once enough staff are present then contextual and organisational decisions must be made.

Non-interventional approach

Some organisations adopt a non-interventional approach in these cases and allow patients to vent their anger on property on the principle that property can be repaired with considerably more ease than humans. Furthermore, in allowing patients to dispel their energy on property, eventually they will tire themselves out and thus be more easily managed. However, some organisations will pursue legal action for financial compensation against patients who destroy hospital property; therefore allowing the patient to continue their destruction does not appear to be operating with the patient's best interests in mind. Similarly, if the property destruction begins to put the patient or others at risk, for example, if electrical wires are being exposed or gas piping torn, then intervention is called for. In this situation, an assessment should be made for the patient's accessibility to weapons. These weapons could be broken furniture, glass, sharp sticks, etc., which would cause considerable damage if they are used.

Team action

In this situation, two or more teams of staff should be amassed with everyone briefed as to their role, function and the target of their action. A spokesperson should attempt to engage the patient in verbal interactions and request a cessation of destruction and a calming down. If the patient can be approached unobtrusively, then this should be done and a 'take-down' can be effected. Unfortunately, this is not always the case and the patient should be approached from several different directions by groups of staff. (In C&R, there is a set procedure, which will not be entered into here as we would like to focus on those staff who are not C&R trained but who may well face these situations.) The spokesperson maintains verbal contact with the patient and attempts to divert their attention away from encroaching staff. The teams of staff should be protected with shields if the patient is throwing, or likely to throw, things at them or will attempt to club members of staff once they are in reach. The shields can be makeshift items such as mattresses, trolleys, chairs, etc., but must be held in such a way that VC can be maintained as the patient is approached. At the prearranged signal, the shields can be used to smother the attack by the patient, then quickly discarded and physical control established. Once the patient is subdued and held appropriately, the move to the next phase can be accomplished.

Attacks on others

Finally, we should note that if a violent person is attacking someone else, then isolating the situation is not appropriate as it leaves the victim at risk. In these situations, the alarm should be raised, support summoned, and one should move straight to physical control as discussed in Chapter 9.

ADVANTAGES AND DISADVANTAGES OF ISOLATION TECHNIQUES

Isolating patients in response to violence and aggression ensures that the damage to others and property is reduced to a minimum. It allows patients time to calm down and regain internal control. The seclusion room can provide patients with a small area which they can master, and it is a place away from the intensity of the ward community (Gutheil 1978). The seclusion room is also said to be a place in which equilibrium can be regained and patients' dignity can be preserved during times of crisis when their behaviour might otherwise cause embarrassment. Isolating patients affords time alone and some space to move in without the emotional impact of human contact (Ray & Rappaport 1995). There are also disadvantages to the use of isolation techniques. Seclusion is said to be a humiliating experience for some (Randell & Walsh 1994) and causes considerable distress (Outlaw & Lowery 1994). During psychiatric crises, patients should not be left alone and human contact is always more desirable than no contact (Stolley 1995). Studies have shown that the mental condition of some patients worsens in seclusion (Mason 1995) and others have indicated that it can be misused as a form of sanction (Mason 1993a).

The advantages and disadvantages can be summarised as seen in Box 8.4.

Box 8.4 Advantages and disadvantages of isolation

Advantages	*Disadvantages*
Damage to others and property is limited	Can be humiliating
Internal control re-established	Causes distress
A space that can be mastered	Human contact is more desirable
Relief from ward intensity	Mental state may worsen
Equilibrium can be regained	Misused as a form of sanction
Dignity can be preserved	Time is distorted

As in all these cases, there is a moral dilemma over which form of control is best used in the crisis moment when one person is attacking another. Isolating patients may, or may not, be deemed better or worse than physically holding them, placing them in mechanical restraints, or giving them medication.

LEGAL CONSIDERATIONS

Although there is no law as such, that pertains directly to the use of isolationary techniques used in psychiatric practice in the UK, there are sufficient legal principles within existing related legislation that can be drawn upon to establish guidelines.

USA

In the USA, the use of seclusion is governed, generally, by state legislation, with most rulings viewing isolation as an emergency psychiatric intervention. However, differences do occur, as evidenced in the Boston State Case of the late 1970s; in this court ruling the judge proclaimed that as the use of seclusion was an emergency measure, the patient could not receive another emergency intervention at the same time (e.g. medication). This caused a great deal of confusion and some considerable debate over the use of isolation techniques as more than just mere restraining devices, with some studies concluding that they were actually treatment modalities (Mason 1994).

UK

In England and Wales, the Mental Health Act Code of Practice (Her Majesty's Stationery Office 1990) states that seclusion is a medical treatment under Section 145 of the Mental Health Act (Her Majesty's Stationery Office 1983; p. 77), but it then informs us that 'seclusion is not a treatment technique and should not feature as part of any treatment programme' (Her Majesty's Stationery Office 1990; p. 77). This, clearly, has led to a great deal of confusion. As there are a number of cases of seclusion being presented before the European Court of Human Rights, it will be interesting to see the legal strategies used by both prosecution and defence, and the reports and related documents that they will draw upon. It is highly likely that the reports from the Royal Colleges of Psychiatrists and Nursing will be used, as will the Health and Safety at Work Act 1990. The latter legislation states that it is the duty of the employer to ensure the provision of a safe working environment.

Possibly the most relevant legislation is Section 5(4) of the Mental Health Act (1983), the nurses' holding power, which, although it does not specifically relate to the use of seclusion, it does allow a patient already in hospital to be immediately restrained for their health or safety, or for the protection of others. The issue of physically restraining someone is fraught with difficulties concerning minimum force, least restrictive measures, technical assault and autonomy, which are dealt with in other chapters of this book. Here, we will briefly mention two points worthy of note in relation to isolating patients rather than physically restraining them. The first involves the notion of illegal confinement, which is the principle at stake in the cases being presented at the European Court. Although patients already in hospital as psychiatric clients may be held against their wishes under the nurses' holding power for 6 hours, in other settings, the person may well not be considered a patient at all, let alone a psychiatric patient (e.g. in casualty departments). The second issue involves inhuman and degrading treatment under Article 3 of the European Convention on Human Rights. However, so far, the European Court has´ not considered seclusion to be a violation of Article 3, although it has considered solitary confinement to be a contravention. The dividing line between the two is fine (Mason 1994).

CONCLUSIONS

In this chapter, we have dealt with the methods of isolating violent and aggressive patients when they become physically combative. There are variations on the theme of seclusion, with various strategies employed to isolate the patient from the remaining ward community that is under threat. The phases of isolation have been outlined, in which the procedure is executed and the patient's responses are assessed. Emergency isolation of patients who are destroying property has been discussed and a strategy for approaching violent patients outlined. There are both advantages and disadvantages to the use of isolation and these have been briefly set out.

Isolating violent and aggressive individuals usually calls for some element of human contact with some degree of force applied. In its raw form, it is the muscular force of the staff pitted against the muscular force of the patient. However, with training, education and practice development, techniques have evolved to ensure that physical restraint is employed in a professional manner with the least pain and injury for all concerned.

9

Physical restraint

KEY POINTS

1. In some cases, defusion attempts fail and physical restraint becomes necessary.
2. Physical restraint is often necessary before other types of restraint can be employed.
3. There are rules of engagement when physical restraint is being applied.
4. There are numerous approaches to physical restraint, including self-defence strategies and Control and Restraint (C&R).
5. Depending upon the patient population, there are other methods of physically restraining someone.

INTRODUCTION

It is often the case that when it has become necessary to restrain a person who has become, or is about to become violent, with the use of either seclusion, emergency medication, or some form of mechanical device, then physical restraint may need to be undertaken as a prerequisite (Mason 1993b). For example, if it is decided to administer a tranquillising drug by intramuscular injection, the patient may need to be physically held whilst this is done. Therefore, physical contact is often necessary when attempting to control violent patients. This contact may well be reactive, for instance, it may take the form of a self-defence technique to fend off blows; or it may be proactive, for instance when one is holding a part of the patient's body. In either event, the important difference between physical restraint and all other types of restraint is that there is human contact between the patient and at least one other person. This human contact has both advantages and disadvantages, which will be spelt out later in this chapter.

Although techniques of physical control exist, their application requires skill to exercise them in a swift and effective manner, and on occasions, this does not always go according to plan and the physical control becomes more a question of muscular force. Similarly, many staff are not trained in a specific technique but rely on learning from others, which has long been a dangerous scenario in terms of the perpetuation of bad practice. This chapter will first deal with the rules of engagement when physically restraining a person; this will also include a brief overview of self-defence strategies and their relationship to the law. Secondly, we will set out the major constructs of C&R, which is the Home Office-approved technique for the management of violence and aggression in prisons. This technique, although originating within the penal system, has now been adopted in, and adapted for, many health care settings. Thirdly, we will outline some other physical restraint techniques that have been reported in the literature; these include gentle holding, bearhugging and pin-down.

RULES OF ENGAGEMENT

There are a number of general principles that ought to guide any action in which physical contact with another human being is going to be undertaken. These include the question of assault, reasonable force, support and time of contact.

Physical contact and assault

First of all, we are all aware of how a comforting arm around the shoulder can emotionally bolster someone who is upset, but technically it can also be an assault, in law. Therefore, we need to define the dangerousness of the behaviours being encountered by specifically identifying the nature of the threat. Once this is clear we have a legal foundation for action. A person may use reasonable force on a person if: 'a breach of the peace is being, or reasonably appears about to be committed ... in common law, this is not only the right of every citizen but it is a duty' (Gostin 1986).

Reasonable force

This brings us to the second principle which is concerned with the notion of reasonable force. Although this is dealt with elsewhere in the book, we will briefly restate the principle here. Dimond (1995) states that: 'reasonableness means, firstly, that force used should be no more than is necessary to accomplish the object for which it is allowed (so retaliation and punishment are not permitted) and secondly, the reaction must be in proportion to the harm which is threatened ... obviously, the greater the severity of the threatened danger, the more reasonable it is to take tougher action'. The major concern in this principle is establishing the balance between the force of the attacker and the response of the defender, and although large displays of imbalances are obvious, from the viewpoint of an observer, it is often difficult to judge the right degree of force to respond with. If the defensive action is believed to be potentially too forceful, then there is a case to be answered in law, and if too weak, then injury, or possibly death, to oneself or others may occur.

Support

The third principle is concerned with support. Only in situations in which life is in immediate danger should a person attempt a physical restraining procedure without summoning help first. In all other cases, it is extremely dangerous to engage a violent person alone; even when being attacked, it is crucial that one calls for help using whatever system is at hand. If no formal alarm system is nearby, then shout as loud as you can.

Time of contact

The final principle to be mentioned refers to the length of time that the aggressor should be physically restrained. Remember that once a physical encounter is exercised, it must have a resolution – that is, a time must come when that physical restraint will have to be released. Therefore, there must be clear objectives about what the physical restraint is to achieve, and what will happen to the patient following the restraint. By establishing this, one can determine the length of time that the person will need to be physically restrained. The principle must be that the person is restrained for the shortest period possible.

Code of practice

As mentioned above, physical restraint involves the use of human beings to apply a bodily force to control another person's behaviour and it is worthwhile reiterating that this must have been preceded by attempts to control the situation with less intrusive methods. Presuming that all other options have failed and that verbal requests have not been responded to, the move to physical control becomes an option (Farrell & Gray 1992). However, before doing so, some further rules of engagement should be considered. First, having summoned help, you are committing others to a physical encounter and clearly are putting them at some, perhaps inevitable, risk. In a recent Department of Health (1997) press release it was stated that: 'staff in the NHS are entitled to feel that they can go about their daily work free from the threat of violence and intimidation', therefore you have a duty to the other staff summoned to ensure the effective and safe management of the violent encounter. Enough staff members should be summoned to deal with the situation but no more than can be effectively managed and communicated with. The restraint procedure will be more effective if it is well planned, with a minimum of well-informed and responsive staff. Second, there is a duty on the part of the health workers to: 'act always in such a manner as to promote and safeguard the interests and well-being of patients and clients' (UKCC 1996). Thus, a quick resolution to the physical restraint is the aim, in order to safeguard the patient and exercise a swift and effective technique by a skilled team.

If circumstances allow, then a briefing session can be used in which the circumstances of the situation can be relayed to other members of the team. Any known relevant history of the aggressor can also be communicated, and staff can be allocated specific tasks for the restraining procedure. Instructions and signals can be quickly rehearsed and if numbers allow, then one staff member should be allocated to be an overall observer of the procedure. This should not be the person in charge but someone independent of the procedure. Large numbers of staff grabbing and scrambling to control a patient can be counterproductive so this should be avoided. A visual check for weapons should be carried out; this may be done discreetly and should include both actual weapons in the possession of the patient and potential weapons in the vicinity. Finally, all others in the area who are not involved in the encounter should be removed from the scene; this includes other patients and visitors, as they provide an audience, which may encourage the aggressor to become more violent. This evacuation should again, be done as discreetly as possible so as not to alarm the aggressor or give prior warning of the intention to take physical control.

A practical guide

Verbal contact with the patient should be maintained prior to, and during, the physical restraint as this will not only help defuse the situation, but will also aid in distracting the person whilst the staff are in preparation. They should empty their pockets, also removing ties, spectacles, badges, pens, etc. and store them safely, as these objects may inadvertently cause injury or be deliberately used by the aggressor as a weapon.

The following guidelines should be observed:

- Once committed to the restraint, move swiftly and decisively as hesitation increases the probability of injury and throws other staff into confusion.

• Do not be distracted from the task that was allocated to you as this will jeopardise others who must cover for the gap.
• When approaching the patient, turn side-on, particularly at close proximity, which will ensure that your front leg forms some protection against a kick to the groin.
• If moving, have your hands ready by your side to be raised in protection or to hold on to the aggressor's arms.
• If standing, touch your chin with the leading hand and rest the other under your elbow. This not only gives the impression of someone who is taking time to think but also puts your arms in a good position to protect against a strike to the head and abdomen.

In establishing physical contact, there are two main strategies depending on whether the patient initiates the contact or whether the staff members do.

Patient-initiated contact

In this situation, the staff members must respond to the events as they occur, which requires speed of thought and speed of action. The commonest events are attacks by the aggressor on another individual. The latter should defend himself by protecting his head and face with either his arms or an appropriate improvised shield (e.g. a chair). The other members of the team should move in and immobilise the patient's limbs. The aggressor can then be lowered to the floor as detailed in the take-down procedure (see p. 136).

Alternatively, and if appropriate, the person under attack may, once a blow has been discharged, bring his arms up deflecting the attacker's arms and move in quickly to restrain the patient by putting his arms around the latter's body. Turning one's face to the side avoids the possibility of being head-butted and drawing one leg up and across the body prevents a knee jab to the groin. Other staff should move in quickly to establish the take-down. Clearly, every situation is different, and therefore, the response to each situation will be different but the simple rule in the event of being attacked is to defend oneself. This may involve using a shield to protect oneself or it may feel more appropriate to move in to restrain the attacker. The individual concerned is the best judge in these circumstances.

Staff-initiated contact

In the situation where the staff members are initiating the physical contact, a signal should be given and those involved should move in quickly to secure their allocated limb and effect the take-down. Again, each situation is different, but a general list of do's and don'ts is outlined in Box 9.1 to provide a guide.

Box 9.1 Some do's and don'ts for physical restraint (adapted from Her Majesty's Stationery Office 1990 and Farrell & Gray 1992)

Do	*Don't*
Make visual check for weapons	Hesitate
Maintain verbal contact	Excessively bend the limbs
Allocate staff to assist and nominate specific tasks	Hit, strike, slap, punch, or kick unless there is imminent threat to life or of serious injury
Employ a briefing session	Intervene on your own unless to preserve life
Commit yourself to the restraint	Place excess weight on any area, especially the patient's neck and stomach
Restrain from behind where possible	Release your hold until safe to do so, and in unison, with a co-ordinated effort, even if the patient says he is now calm
Remove contents of pockets, ties, spectacles, etc.	
Remain calm	
Employ a firm tone of voice	
Protect the patient's head and vulnerable spots	
Remove the patient's shoes when down	
Hold the main limbs near the joints to prevent excessive leverage	
If alone, safeguard yourself and summon support	
Avoid holding the patient's neck	

CRISIS INTERVENTION

When engaged in an aggressive encounter, we should always be aware that no technique is totally without risks and that things can unexpectedly go wrong. Furthermore, we may come under specific attack ourselves and need to take defensive action in order to safeguard ourselves. The remainder of this chapter will outline some recognised approaches to responding to being attacked and physically intervening to control an assailant.

Self-defence techniques

Rice et al (1989) have outlined a self-defence against assault programme that is taught in Ontario, Canada. This programme encompasses eight broad areas:

1. Stance – the basic stance is as we have outlined above, but there is additional advice given about not standing like a 'prizefighter' and never turning one's back on an aggressive individual.
2. Grabbing attacks – there are six general grabbing-type attacks that the aggressor may use; a list of these is shown in Box 9.2.
3. Striking attacks – generally speaking, these are of two types. The first includes punching-type attacks. These are usually aimed at the head, in

Box 9.2 Types of grabbing attack

Type of Attack	*Response*
One-hand cross-grab, in which the aggressor grabs your right hand with his right hand (or left with left)	The grabbed arm should be kept bent with the thumb upwards, clasp both hands for added strength. Rotate the arms making a circular movement. This should dislodge the grab. Alternatively, bring your hands swiftly upwards to your shoulder, which should have the same effect
Two-hand cross-grab, whereby the aggressor grabs both of your wrists with both of his hands	Move your hands in and out in an irregular fashion briskly, whilst travelling backwards with your back straight. According to Rice et al (1989), this confuses the patient and breaks his hold
Front-hand choke, when the patient clutches your throat with both of his hands	Clasp your hands together linking them through one of his arms. Raise one of your elbows above his elbow and lower your other elbow below his other one. Then quickly reverse this position keeping your hands tightly clasped, so that the arm above his is yanked downwards and the one below his is pushed upwards. This should dislodge the choke
Rear-hand choke, where the patient grabs your throat from behind with both of his hands	Raise one of your arms high in the air and quickly rotate whilst stepping forwards. This should break the choke
Hair grab from the rear	Place both of your hands on the hands of the attacker who has grabbed your hair so as to cap them. Pull them tight to your head. Rotate to face the patient whilst at the same time dropping your head, and move in closer to the attacker. This will twist his wrist and arm thus dislodging his grip on your hair
Rear choke, with the arm across your throat (this is possibly the most dangerous of all non-weapon attacks)	Rice et al recommend tucking your chin into his arm and biting it if possible. If not, then pull the choking arm away as much as possible and rotate your neck towards the wrist of the choking arm to release some pressure on your carotid artery and trachea. Then step to the side whilst blocking the patient's heel with your foot and convert the choke to a headlock. This will further release the pressure on your neck. Release can now be effected by either grabbing the attacker's groin (if male) or by moving backward, briskly, whilst at the same time pulling sharply downwards on the arm that is holding you

which case, they may come from a fair distance – that is, wild swings with the attacker's fist travelling in an arc from around his side. The defence for this is to raise both hands close together with the arms bent and move into the swing of the patient's arm. However, if the patient is close in, then the punches are usually short jabs to the body rather than the head. Blows of this type can be blocked by lowering one's elbows into the path of the strike. The second includes kicking-type attacks and the most frequent are front kicks to the groin. If you are close, then move even closer whilst at the same time twisting to the side and bringing your knee upwards, and across your body, to present your leg as a shield. If there is a greater distance between you and the kicker then turn to the side, step backwards as he kicks, and either knock his kicking leg away with your forward hand or grab his leg from underneath and restrain him.

4. Biting attacks – as Rice et al (1989) point out, these attacks are particularly unpleasant. In these situations do not pull away from the bite as this will make things worse; instead push the part that is being bitten hard into the patient's mouth, grab his nostrils and close them. This will often succeed in the release of the bite as the assailant opens his mouth to breathe. Alternatively, press your middle knuckle of each hand (one if you cannot manage both) under the biter's ears.

5. Weapons – we will deal with this more fully in Chapter 12. However, Rice et al have some excellent advice on these situations; they suggest that 'if possible, run away' (Rice et al 1989, p. 142). The main defence against assault by a weapon is to arm yourself with a defensive weapon. This may be a chair, a cushion, a trolley, or even a belt with a buckle spun fast to keep the assailant at bay. Failing the acquisition of a defensive weapon, keep moving by bobbing and weaving to keep your distance from the weapon. Do not try anything heroic, and escape as soon as you can.

6. Offence – as mentioned above, an attacker should not be struck unless there is an imminent life-threatening situation. However, Rice et al (1989), whilst agreeing that patients should not be struck unless there is imminent danger, also suggest that this can be extended to include situations when there are no safer alternatives. If a strike has to be undertaken, then a sharp blow, or strong push, to the solar plexus is the preferred method; note, however, that although this is usually quite safe if undertaken correctly, if the target is missed, there could be damage to the ribs. Another defensive strategy is the 'equalization technique' (Rice et al 1989) in which the defender lies on his back and rapidly kicks at the attacker with alternating feet. Should the assailant move around the defender, then the latter can quickly swivel on his back to maintain his kicking feet at the aggressor.

7. Intervening in others' fights – do not get between fighting persons of any description, as you are likely to become the target of both. Instead, first

command them to stop fighting immediately, and if that does not work, or you have not got time as someone is being injured, then come up behind the dominant aggressor and push (not kick) one of your feet behind one of his knees to collapse him. At the same time, pull his collar backwards and catch him as he falls backwards, lowering him to the floor.

8. Falls – during aggressive encounters, falling over is a very common experience and it is important to attempt to avoid becoming injured as a result of the fall. Rice et al suggest that when falling forward, keep the knees and body straight and break the fall with your outstretched, and slightly bent, arms. The face should be turned to one side. When moving and falling forwards or to the side, the knees should be bent and one hand lowered to the floor with the elbow bent, converting the forward movement of the fall into a forward roll. If falling backward, then bend the neck forward looking down your body, keep stepping backwards for as long as you are able during which time you will be getting closer to the ground. Break the fall with your hands and let yourself roll as far as the momentum will take you. If you are travelling fast, then you may need to convert the fall into a backward roll over your shoulder to avoid hurting your head and neck.

There is a lack of empirical evidence on whether attendance on such courses as those mentioned here actually prevents violence and aggression occurring or simply manages it in such a way that injuries are decreased. However, one study worthy of note is that by Phillips & Rudestam (1995). These authors reported on the effect of non-violent self-defence training on male psychiatric staff members' aggression and fear, and found that: 'behaviourally expressed fear and aggression were significantly reduced among staff who received both didactic and physical skills training' (Phillips & Rudestam 1995, p. 164). In the other two groups they studied, didactic training only and no training at all, they found no significant changes in these items.

Control and Restraint (C&R)

As in the teaching programme outlined in the previous section from the study of Rice et al (1989), we do not suggest that this text replace attendance on recognised courses; in fact quite the reverse, we strongly recommend participation on quality courses. We outline the above approaches to offer the reader supportive material so that they may make informed choices. In this section, we will now give a broad overview of C&R and its developments.

The issue of staff safety in health care facilities became a major agenda issue in the USA before it did in the UK, probably because of the extent of litigation exercised in the USA. Therefore, it is not surprising that

C&R has its roots in defensive methods of managing violence and aggression in institutions in the USA. In fact the similarities between C&R and the self-defence techniques reported by Rice et al (1989) above are remarkable. The UK government department, the Home Office, first approved the C&R course for use in the Prison Service in the late 1970s, following which, it was adopted in special hospitals in the wake of the Richie report on a case of death in seclusion in Broadmoor. Thereafter, it was used in parts of the National Health Service (NHS) for the control of violence in health care settings. As a recognised course, it is becoming increasingly more important, as health authorities attempt to equip staff to manage escalating amounts of aggression in many areas of health care.

As a product of that demand, C&R has evolved to meet the needs of some facilities that have a particular difficulty with the terms 'control' and 'restraint', and have mutated the terms to 'care' and 'responsibility'. The differences are minimal but C&R has expanded on other options available in the management of violence and aggression prior to the crisis emerging. C&R provides a framework of practical skills, with a level of team work, with the aim that nobody is hurt, before or during, the combative crisis. The idea underpinning C&R is that, in the rare circumstances when the only option left is to restrain an aggressor physically, the restrainers operate according to a prescribed action and can function effectively as a three-person team. This means that people who have completed the course can actively assess the situation and will make informed, calculated decisions during this crucial time. Guidance is given on how restraint should be executed, who is in charge of decision making and who activates the commands.

C&R is taught by approved trainers. The length of the course varies depending on the needs of the group being trained, but is generally between a day and a week or so, with follow-up refresher training at specified points. The courses also introduce de-escalatory skills so that the students are clear about the principle of C&R only as a last resort option.

Thereafter, C&R training follows both a theoretical and a practical course, addressing physical restraint issues that require the students to work through potential scenarios with the use of role play, correction and reflection. It is often the case that one individual student will play the part of the aggressor whilst others take responsibility for the attempted diffusion, followed by the safe and effective resolution of the hostile situation. The training involves using breakaway techniques, and immobilising the patient with and without the use of a shield.

Breakaway techniques

An important part of the course is dedicated to what are termed 'breakaway techniques'; these help the victim to neutralise the hostile confrontation and make an escape. The breakaway techniques are useful for the most common one-on-one attacks. They involve a variety of simple moves that incorporate leverage rather than strength, which means that relatively weak individuals can disengage a variety of the common holds used by a stronger aggressor, thus leaving the intended victim to flee the dangerous situation. In summary, these manoeuvres will help when being:

- held by the hair
- grabbed by the neck or shoulders, from both the front and rear
- strangled
- held at a point around the chest or abdomen.

In addition, the training provides the student with practical steps that will also temporarily divert or distract the aggressor's attention so that an escape can be achieved. This can include techniques such as:

1. Thumb release – this is used on a fist that is clutching accessible clothing or parts of the body. The bent thumb is pushed down at the finger nail to disengage the attacker and effect an escape.
2. The straight arm hold – this manoeuvre utilises the aggressor's arm. The elbow is locked so the arm is held in a straight position and may then be used as a lever. One hand holds the aggressor's wrist area and the other applies a controlled force to the back of the middle/upper arm. The aggressor can then be controlled and moved to the floor, providing time to move away.
3. The sternum technique – this involves employing a knuckle to the sternum of the aggressor and using either controlled twisting or rigorous moving; this causes a sharp pain and the aggressor is diverted and moves away.
4. The knuckle diversion – this involves rigorous movement of the knuckle to the back of the grabbing hand causing temporary pain, again forcing diversion and release.

Immobilising the patient

The skills and resources required for immobilisation fall into two broad categories: (a) immobilising the unarmed person, and (b) immobilising the person who has a weapon.

Immobilisation is effected by a three-person team who approach the aggressor swiftly with one staff member leading and the other two tucked in behind in a side-on position. The objective is to immobilise the aggressor safely (usually taking him to the floor in a controlled manner) and this is achieved by the lead person holding the head, whilst the other two team members take responsibility for holding an arm each in a secure position. The moves are performed while one person talks calmly and clearly to the aggressor in an attempt to de-escalate the situation. One at a time, each arm is secured in a hold. Once this has been achieved then pressure can be applied at the wrists to gain cooperation. Thereafter, the holds may be released or maintained depending on the behaviour of the aggressor.

Safety equipment

Safety of all is a central consideration, so if the patient is armed (firearms excluded), the team should defuse the situation whilst wearing safety equipment that may include padding around limbs, helmets and shields. The strategies used follow the same basic format as for the unarmed situation. The shields in this situation are central to defending oneself as the situation is being brought under control. The shields are also used to impede the aggressor's movements. Part of C&R training teaches staff members how to use a shield and other protective equipment effectively as part of a team to defend themselves from thrown items and to immobilise an extremely violent individual. In this, the staff rush into the situation at a predetermined time in a choreographed, coordinated manner, protected by the shields; these also hinder the patient's ability to swing his arms and legs, as the shields are placed against his body. Rapidly, the aggressor finds himself between a natural surface (wall or floor) and the C&R team shields. It is at this point that C&R holds are applied and the situation is brought under control.

Also incorporated in the training, is the preparation of staff in moving the violent individual from one place to another; this is given in the form of escort training. It enables an aggressor to be moved safely with the use of the C&R team approach.

Advantages and disadvantages

The use of C&R in health care settings can give entirely the wrong impression about the care delivery being offered. However, it provides a systematic and expansive method that incorporates a variety of options for the management of the violent or potentially violent person. At the centre of criticism about it, is the debate over the administration of pain to control the violent individual. Some argue that this is a result of the aggressor dispensing his own pain, fighting against the holds, whilst others suggest it is the restrainers applying an element of force that causes the pain. Suffice to say that, as with any physical restraint, dangers do exist. Clearly, control by others, particularly over prolonged periods, can be counterproductive and even dangerous in some instances. Readers need to be aware that each patient's physical condition requires careful assessment prior to any combative behaviour, and subsequent physical restraint to assure that manoeuvres or whole techniques will not exacerbate injuries or aggravate physical conditions. Box 9.3 is a short summary of the advantages and disadvantages of the use of C&R.

Box 9.3 Advantages and disadvantages of the use of C&R

Advantages	*Disadvantages*
Achieves a disciplined and controlled response to an aggressor	Oppressive and can be overcontrolling
Provides suitable training for staff managing violent situations	Can be mechanistic and inappropriate with some populations in some contexts
Aimed at minimising risk of injury to all parties	Can be misused as the first option, rather than the last resort
Provides for an identified leader and clear role delineation	Has a macho image
Increases staff confidence to manage violence	Requires a team of three people
Manoeuvres, holds and strategies are formally taught on approved courses	Overzealous use will cause pain increasing likelihood of further aggression
Measured response	Uses pain to control
Physical injury less likely	Requires regular training updates

OTHER APPROACHES

It would be wrong, and bordering on asinine, to suggest that a specific type of physical restraint, or indeed any other form of controlling measure, is suitable for all people, on all occasions and in all situations. Although some commentators are confident enough to claim that a particular practice should never be used, the word 'never' is too final in the world of management of violence and aggression. The authors' position is that the response to violence and aggression should, as we have pointed out previously, take into consideration the person, the place and the circumstances, and be the minimum required to control the aggressor safely. The small aggressive child with learning difficulties may require one level of restraint but when that child grows to an adult and remains aggressive, he may need a completely different level of response. However, the common theme throughout these levels is the notion of human touch – the physical contact between two or more individuals. Touch is a concept that we are all familiar with and we recognise its importance in rearing children, as well as in our own personal relationships. Furthermore, we recognise the difference between the human contact that is made, to say, safeguard someone from danger and contact that is designed to cause pain. Yet it is through the touch that the messages of pain, pleasure or protection are transmitted, as Tronick (1995) put it: 'touch conveys specific messages … for example, certain forms of touch, … might convey the message "you are safe" whereas other forms of touch … may convey the message "you are physically threatened"' (p. 54). Therefore, the context and manner in which physical restraint is conducted, are crucially important in transmitting the appropriate message.

We would now like to deal with some forms of touch in relation to physically restraining someone. Although for ease of dealing with these techniques we have sectioned them into subdivisions, which gives the impression of clearly delineated procedures, note that in reality, there is a great deal of overlap between them.

Gentle holding

Gentle holding is part of the wider concept of 'gentle teaching' whereby the carer remains warm, compassionate and positive whilst loosely restraining and guiding the disturbed patient. The fundamental principle of gentle holding is as a physical intervention to eliminate undesirable problem behaviours without the use of punishment procedures. Grounded in this, is the concept of social reinforcement with an overall aim of conveying to the patient a clear positive regard in response to their expression of negative behaviours. The patient is allowed some free movement of the limbs but for the safety of all concerned, is gently restrained within certain parameters (Gates, Wray & Newell 1996). It is rooted in the idea that the person is considered valuable and worthwhile, irrespective of the behaviours that are currently being emitted. It is said to allow health workers to see people as they really are (Crowhurst, Carlile & Horsfall 1993).

The gentle holding procedure is more successful when the aggression is diffuse, as in a temper tantrum where the lashing out is non-directive and random. However, it is less likely to be successful when aggression is focused and directed at a specific individual. Conceptually, random aggression usually represents a release valve for the dissipation of pent-up anger or frustrations, whereas, targeted violence usually implies a more structured and motivational scenario.

Gentle holding is also concerned with guiding a person's behaviour in the form of structuring his movements without totally restraining them, as one would do, say, in an epileptic seizure where the movements of the limbs are uncontrolled and may well cause injury to the patient or to others unless he is guided safely. Gentle holding is geared towards children with learning difficulties and may not be appropriate in other spheres of health care.

Natural therapeutic holding

This technique, as outlined by Stirling & McHugh (1997), was developed out of dissatisfaction with the more formal C&R outlined above. As in gentle holding, it is grounded in a positive regard for the patient and seeks to readdress the aversive techniques that other strategies employ. It is reported to be non-punitive and painless, and appears far less domineering than C&R. The basis of this type of holding is the establishment of clear therapeutic goals and is concerned with the patient learning from the experience.

Thus far, it has been used in 'a small community residential service for people with learning disabilities' (Stirling & McHugh 1997; p. 304), and it may well be restricted to this type of client group. However, it would seem important that its application is tested in other settings and with a wider population before conclusions can be drawn.

Holding therapy

Holding Therapy may well be little different from the natural therapeutic holding mentioned above but we feel that it deserves to be somewhat differentiated, as the literature suggests that it is used on a rather more aggressive patient population. It has been reported in Germany as an effective method for 'omnipotent (tyrannical) children' (Burchard 1988, p. 89) and in the USA on 'seriously disturbed violent adolescents (aged 12–19 years) on an inpatient psychiatric unit' (Miller, Walker & Friedman 1989). The 'holding' comprises the physical control of the person's limbs by carers who maintain contact with the disturbed person for as long as it takes for him to calm down. Again, a major concern is with the positive regard and attitude of the person(s) doing the holding, which purportedly gives it its therapeutic substance. The external control (the positive holding) is maintained until the disturbed person regains internal control and equilibrium. External control is maintained by holding the person's arms to a fixed point, which could be the arms of a chair or the person's side. It has also been used in family therapy situations where family members have been taught how to effect the technique when the family member becomes disturbed (Vorster 1990). The advantage of this being that it is more natural for family members to hold their child than it is for the therapist.

Bearhugging

This technique probably draws all the above themes together in an informal way. The procedure is generally used on children but can be employed on adolescents and possibly some adult populations. The disturbed person is approached from behind and the carer places their arms around him in a bearhug. The carer's head is placed next to the aggressor's head and side-of-face to side-of-face contact is maintained with gentle pressure so that the disturbed person cannot headbutt either backwards or sidewards into the carer's face. The advantages of this position is that the contact can be firm enough to maintain control, can be released gently as calm ensues, and the carer can talk quietly to the patient, reassuring him. The bearhug position is in other contexts, one of a friendly and intimate nature, so if undertaken in a positive therapeutic manner in the disturbed situation, it can convey not only messages of control, but also those of a compassionate nature.

Pin-down

We would like to finish this section with a few words on pin-down, which is a technique that was developed mainly for use with disturbed children in residential social service settings. The method originated as a means of holding down disturbed aggressive children by controlling all four limbs, which were held fast until the person became calm. However, it developed incrementally to include a regimen of sanctions that, in some circumstances, involved stripping the child, holding beyond calming him as a form of punishment, and removing certain privileges as a sanction. Clearly, this was unethical and unprofessional; in the UK in 1990, it led to an inquiry with the result that it was ultimately outlawed (Baldwin & Barker 1995). This is a good, but sad, example of how a recognised technique of restraint can develop, through bad practice and lack of personal and professional scrutiny, into abuse.

CONCLUSIONS

In the management of violence and aggression, the images that are evoked are usually unpleasant, in that the violence and aggression exercised by the perpetrator is disturbing, and the use of force to quell the violence can often be equally unpleasant (Maier & Van Rybroek 1990). When violence occurs and others are involved in controlling it, this must be a question of one, or more, persons dominating the will of another (the aggressor). Although we can encompass this control within therapeutic paradigms such as therapeutic holding or we can mutate the semantics of C&R to become care and responsibility, none the less, it remains the domination of one person's will by that of another. Although one can aim for it to be in the interests of the recipient, with the best of intentions and operated within a professional framework, yet the fundamental principle of control is inescapable.

This chapter has focused on physical restraint, whereby the human contact between those involved is the basis of the controlling procedure. All these methods utilise human force to control another individual. From setting out the 'rules of engagement', we have outlined a self-defence programme aimed at the management of violence and aggression. C&R has also been reviewed in relation to its advantages and disadvantages, and finally other approaches have been briefly highlighted. In all these approaches, the physical holding and control of disturbed people was pivotal in preventing harm. However, our implicit themes are that the holding is for very short periods and that the disturbed individual quickly regains self-control. However, this does not cover every case, as some individuals are chronically assaultive and may require other forms of restraint. We therefore now turn our attention to controlling measures that use some form of equipment, which we refer to as mechanical restraints.

Note:
The discussion of the techniques in this chapter in no way replaces attendance on recognised courses. Course attendance and practical demonstration and application of the methods by qualified instructors are strongly recommended before any of these techniques are applied.

10

Mechanical control

KEY POINTS

1. Mechanical restraints have been refined over the past 2 decades.
2. They are considered preferable to other forms of restraint by some mental health workers.
3. There are a number of legal concerns regarding the use of mechanical restraints.
4. The prime negative aspect of the use of mechanical restraints is the visual image that they produce.
5. Some modern mechanical restraints are customised for individual needs.

INTRODUCTION

In the last chapter we discussed the crisis of combat in which the aggressive person becomes actually assaultive, and the fact that in that phase of the attack, some method of physical restraint is required. In response to such attacks, in the name of self-defence or the protection of others, we saw how 'hands-on' physical control could be established, with the safety of all concerned in mind. Once physical contact is established, there are serious legal and ethical considerations that must be borne in mind and govern our action in such difficult moments of crisis. Clearly, these considerations restrict and limit our interventions to ensure that the minimum force is used in the least restrictive manner. Yet, despite this, injuries can be sustained by both staff and patients, and no matter which method of physical holding is used, the sight of one or more persons controlling and dominating another human being, jars one's sensibilities. There can be few people who have not, at one time or another in their lives, attempted to intervene in a fight to prevent one person from assaulting another. Whether it be in the playground or on the sports field, most readers will remember physically holding an aggressive person and trying to reason with them. The sight of such brawls, or attempts to control them, are images which few like to see; however, most people recognise the need to intervene to prevent injury. Mechanical restraints share a similar position for mental health workers in psychiatric practice.

The term 'mechanical' is loosely associated with 'manacle', both of which conjure up images of rattling chains against old stone walls in some dreary, dank, dungeon in medieval times. Furthermore, 'mechanical' also gives an impression of cold steel machine parts operating without thought or feelings, merely going through the motions, in a set predetermined manner. However, as with many other aspects of psychiatric practice, developments since the Dark Ages have taken place, and even since the Second World War, progress has been made, albeit often slowly. Just as psychosurgical techniques, psychotropic medications and psychoanalytic interventions have developed from often crude beginnings to more refined levels of operation, mechanical restraints of today are subtly different from the shackles of the past. It is fair to say that fundamentally, they fulfil the same function, but at least in terms of compassionate management, they are of a different ilk at the turn of the 21st century. For example, they are usually specially designed and custom made for each individual's requirement. They are generally made of leather and allow for some degree of freedom of movement. The cold, manacled chains of the past have, rightly, gone the way of trephining, shock treatment and purging.

One aspect which has changed little over the years, however, is the offensiveness of the image of fellow human beings with their movements restricted by some form of restraining equipment. In an article by Maier & Van Rybroek (1990) about the issue of offensive images, they pointedly note that 'managing aggression isn't pretty' (p. 357). In this short article, their concern is with the old debate as to which form of restraint is least unacceptable and they ponder as to whether using seclusion is an easier option because it is a case of 'out of sight is out of mind'. They suggest that this is a form of denial that is more difficult to engage in when a person is in mechanical restraints as the sight is visually more unpleasant. They conclude: 'we look forward to the day when the image of an aggressive patient in ambulatory restraints will be as acceptable as the surgical patient attached to an IV pole or an adolescent wearing [dental] braces' (Maier & Van Rybroek 1990, p. 357).

ISSUES OF PRAGMATISM

From the literature there appears to be two main patient populations to which mechanical restraints are applied: elderly agitated, and violent psychiatric patients. The elderly agitated tend to have soft restraints, protection nets and various devices to limit their movements, whereas violent psychiatric patients are more inclined to have several point restraints, Posey belts (see p. 170) and ambulatory restraints. In both groups, there tends to be a chronic pattern of problematic behaviour before a decision is taken to use mechanical restraints. Violent psychiatric patients are likely to have had a long and chequered history of violent attacks with many staff injuries sustained along the way. They are also likely to have some form of organic impairment as well as psychic dysfunction, and be unresponsive to treatment. They have usually had long periods of institutional care and there are major considerations as to their quality of life. They are usually considered too assaultive for special observations or physical holding.

Staff managing violent and aggressive patients in diverse mental health settings are prone to attack on a potentially constant basis (Whittington & Wykes 1992) which, irrespective of assault frequency, causes nursing staff some degree of stress. The stress can be divided into acute and chronic types. In acute stress, this occurs as an adrenaline rush of violent incidents happening when an actual assault is ongoing or has just taken place. In this phase, the state of arousal from such acute stress, although usually relatively short lived, is predominantly high. However, in chronic stress there is often little real awareness of either the source of stress or the response to it. In this phase, there may also be little conscious awareness of the continuing daily stress of working in these environments between the acute phases of assaults and the chronic phases of attack-free periods. Daily life goes on without major incidents but always with the potential for attack. The environments may be tense and hostile with considerable verbal aggression, stalking or pacing, which creates fear and foreboding. This is an extremely unhealthy working environment and by no means can it be considered fit for staff or therapeutic for patients. Such chronic stress can have serious deleterious consequences on the long-term well-being of staff and other patients, and can also lead to the development of aberrant ward/unit cultures (Caudill et al 1952; Richman 1998). These may include the ward staff responding to the 'tradition of toughness' (Morrison 1990) and the underreporting of assaults as the latter become part of 'normalised' behaviour (Lion, Snyder & Merrill 1981).

Mechanical restraint versus chemical and isolation methods

The response to chronically assaultive patients usually involves high dosages of medication, long periods of isolation, or some form of mechanical restraint and, in some cases, a combination of all three. Although there is contention about the moral implications of all these types of interventive modalities, certain units, hospitals and countries tend to favour one over the other. Arguments abound as to the drugged-up and zombified (medication), isolated and abandoned (secluded), and undignified and trussed-up (restrained) patients (Mason 1993c,d). Whatever emotive terms are used to emphasise a particular point of view, there is no categorical moral imperative regarding the propriety, or otherwise, of any of these techniques. However, it is fair to say that, for whatever reasons, there is more use of mechanical restraints in the USA and some European countries than in the UK, where seclusion and medication, rather than mechanical restraints, are favoured for chronically assaultive patients at the point of crisis.

As mentioned above, the debate on the use of mechanical restraints for those patients who are extremely violent, pivots upon which method is viewed as the least objectionable. Bearing in mind that we are focusing upon patients who are chronically assaultive over long periods of time and who have not responded to treatment interventions, the question of control is a central issue. When in the throes of attack, as we have seen in earlier chapters, the person must be restrained from causing injury to others. Therefore, whether one prefers quick-acting medication, isolation, physical holding or a mechanical restraint, depends upon an individual assessment of the moral implications of each. However, it is difficult to try to reveal the constructs underlying this morality. Let us take as an example of a person who becomes violent and 30 minutes later is immobilised; the patient's inability to make a further attack is due to one of the following reasons:

1. medication has tranquillised him
2. several staff are holding him fast in C&R holds
3. he is alone in a seclusion room
4. his arms are held in a waist belt.

The question for readers is 'which one is least unacceptable?', Or, put another way, 'which one would readers prefer for themselves should they need to be immobilised to prevent them attacking another person?'

There are, of course, no right or wrong answers to this. However, we suggest that the answer the reader makes to the first question is likely to relate to how the patient *looks*, the second question relates to how you would *feel*. There is evidence to suggest that the acceptability factor is more concerned with the visual imagery that it produces than it is to do with any moral interpretation of least restrictive practice, safety or dignity.

McDonell, Sturmey & Dearden (1993) reported on a study in which subjects were shown video sequences of three restraining techniques used on an aggressor. Although only tentative conclusions were drawn, they did show that subjects preferred a restraint procedure that involved sitting the patient in a chair rather than one that involved lying him on the floor. They also emphasised an important point by distinguishing between the acceptability of a restraining procedure and its effectiveness. Often a procedure may be effective but not acceptable, while some interventions may be acceptable but not effective. It is in the middle ground between acceptability and effectiveness that the law operates.

LEGAL CONSIDERATIONS

American legislation

Elyn Saks (1986) set out the main principles of American legislation pertaining to the use of mechanical restraint. He noted that liberty is central to American jurisprudence, from which the use of mechanical restraints deviates. American patients have the right to choose which treatments they will and will not have, except in the case of an emergency. Violence to others by psychiatric patients is considered to be such an emergency. The principles underlying US law are, first, that a person should be deprived of liberty only when presenting a serious risk of harm to self or others, second, that the extent of the deprivation of liberty should be that necessary to achieve safety and no more, third, that the patient should choose the restraint wherever possible, and fourth, that the infringement on the patient's liberty should be the absolute minimum required. However, use of mechanical restraint in America departs from these principles, according to Saks (1986) as: 'most states allow hospital staff to put patients in restraints when there is no serious threat of injury and without any clear showing of their efficacy' (p. 1841). Saks proceeded to outline the fundamental problem of whether mechanical restraint should be considered as a therapeutic enterprise or as a management technique. He highlighted the differences between American and British experiences of using mechanical restraint, and claimed a degree of success in Britain for, generally, avoiding the use of these restraints for all, but the most seriously violent patients.

British legislation

If liberty is a central tenet of American society, then reasonableness is the British equivalent. This includes reasonableness in terms of both how feasible it is for professionals to predict violence and foresee harm to the patient or others, and how reasonable the restraint is to prevent such injury. Dimond (1995) claims that: 'reasonableness means, firstly, that the force used should be no more than is necessary to accomplish the object for which it is allowed (so retaliation, revenge and punishment are not permitted) and, secondly, the reaction must be in proportion to the harm which is threatened' (p. 200). Dimond goes on to recommend that the circumstances, or context, in which the violence occurs must be taken into consideration. This context includes the strength, size and expertise of the attacker as well as that of the defendant. Clearly, an increased degree of danger allows for a greater degree of force used for protection and the law takes into consideration the fact that, in some circumstances, the defender may have only a brief moment of time to make up his mind.

The notion of minimum, or reasonable, force in British common law is closely related to the American equivalent of least restrictive alternative (LRA) when discussed in relation to mental health practice. Reasonable force is a concept that requires practitioners to apply no more restraint than is necessary to accomplish the task to which it is being applied, and should be proportionate to the danger that is confronted in both degree and duration (Dimond 1995). The least restrictive alternative has its roots in a 1960 US Supreme Court case (Gutheil, Appelbaum & Wexler 1983) in which the principle was laid down that mentally disabled persons have the right to treatment in the least confining manner (Fisher et al 1995).

Both the British and American principles have difficulties for practising clinicians. The problems involve the accuracy of assessment of the required amount of force, which is notoriously difficult to ascertain. If too much force or restriction is applied, then there are professional and legal repercussions, whereas if too little force is exercised, then injuries may be sustained. Furthermore, once restrictions are applied, the question of duration features large and with similar problems (e.g. too long or not long enough). This legal perspective can be countered, to some degree, by the production of guidelines. (An example of these will be presented later in the chapter.)

TYPES OF MECHANICAL RESTRAINT

The first thing to note about the use of mechanical restraints is the wide variety of apparatuses employed to restrict a person's movements. Some of these are quite subtle but the majority are stark and undiscerning, some are used legitimately whilst others are employed illicitly, some are used in the interests of staff and others are used in the interests of the patient, and some are used to stop the patient attacking themselves whilst others are adopted to protect others. The second thing to observe is the wide range of clinical conditions in which they are employed, from children with learning difficulties to elderly agitated senile patients, and from the psychiatrically disturbed to the severely intoxicated. The ingenuity of the human mind to invent mechanisms of control is surpassed only by its ability to devise methods of destruction. Before concentrating on the specific mechanical restraints used for chronically violent adults who are psychiatrically disturbed, we would like to mention briefly some of the methods that are used on other patient populations.

In an excellent article, which has not lost any of its potency for being almost 30 years old, Dewhurst (1970) outlined some interesting methods of restraint (that is, if by restraint one means some piece of apparatus that is applied to restrict the patient's movements).

The 'Mussadiq manoeuvre'. The first restraint was the 'Mussadiq manoeuvre' in which patients' day clothes are removed and they are given night clothes to wear. This is named after the Persian Prime Minister, Mussadiq, who attended crisis meetings clad in pyjamas, possibly to gain sympathy. It is used in some psychiatric establishments to deter absconders.

ECT. The second of Dewhurst's restraints was the 'electric sledge-hammer', he was referring here to the excessive use of electroconvulsive therapy (ECT). Although writing at a time when ECT was, perhaps, used more widely than it is today, the interesting point is that it was a legitimate psychiatric intervention interpreted by him as a rather crude method of restraint.

The Buxton chair. The third method of restraint was the Buxton chair for the elderly confused patient. This chair was usually on wheels and had a mechanism that allowed it to tip back, making egress from the chair difficult; a tray would also be fixed in front of the seated person to prevent him moving forwards out of the chair. There have been consistent reports of the continued use of this method of restraint up to the present day (Harris 1996).

Restraints for mentally impaired patients

Other types of restraint we would mention are the various apparatuses used mainly for mentally impaired patients. For example:

- Singh, Dawson & Manning (1981) reported on a profoundly impaired patient who would engage in face slapping and punching, and who was placed in a jacket with arms that could be tied behind the back.
- An autistic person who hit out, kicked and pulled hair and who was tethered by the wrists or ankles to a chair whilst sitting, or a bed when prone (Mattson & Keyes 1988).
- Foam-padded gloves and an American-style football helmet were used on a profoundly impaired person who engaged in head banging, hand biting and placing fingers in his eye sockets (Dorsey et al 1982).
- A clear plastic spherical bubble helmet was placed over the head of an autistic person who engaged in self-biting of the arms and hands (Neufeld & Fantuzzo 1984).
- Oven mitts were placed on the hands of a profoundly impaired person who constantly placed his hands in his mouth (Mazaleski et al 1994).

From this brief and limited review, we can see that for almost every type of disorder there is some form of apparatus that can be innovatively adopted in an attempt to control the behaviour of the disturbed person.

Many mechanical restraints have been created as a direct response to specific problems from specific individuals. Unfortunately, this can result in illicit practices as well as quite legitimate ones. It is not unknown for an elderly confused patient to have his dressing gown belt tied around a chair to stop him from getting up, or a flailing patient to have his hand bandaged to a cot-side. What makes these practices illegal is not so much their action but the lack of legitimation and sanction. Someone who is attempting to pull his eyes out may well have boxing gloves fitted as a temporary measure to stop him, but this needs the sanction of multidisciplinary teams, the patient's relatives and ethics committees, as well as some involvement with the Mental Health Act Commission and patient advocacy services.

As was said earlier, many of today's modern restraining devices are customised and made for individual cases, therefore attempting to categorise them is difficult. However, some grouping is possible under the following headings:

1. restraints of the arms
2. restraints of the legs
3. total body restraints
4. bed restraints
5. mouth restraints
6. ambulatory restraints

Restraints of the arms

The main type of hand and arm restraint is the Posey belt or shirt, from the American Posey Company. The belt is made of leather and approximately 15 cm wide; it is fastened around the violent person's waist, and the other end attached to a bed. The shirt is a full garment with the hands suitably restrained. There are many variations to this theme, including abdominal belts that can be fastened to a fixed point and various straps that can be used to restrain the violent attacker. In some cases, these can be located on an actual chair fixed down in a given area (e.g. a restraining room or a van for transporting violent persons). There are also safety vests, which are similar to the old straitjackets in holding the arms within the garment, thus restricting the patient from striking out (Fig. 10.1). Other garments include the 'poncho' type, which fits over the head and can be drawn down over the arms of the attacker. Finally, there are a number of belt types that function to restrain the arms. These include the chest belt, which fixes the upper arm leaving the lower arm and hands with limited movement, and the pelvic belt, which holds the lower arms to the sides. In some instances these belts have cuffs attached to the sides of the webbing in which the wrists are placed. The violent person, thus, cannot raise the hands to strike out (Fig. 10.2).

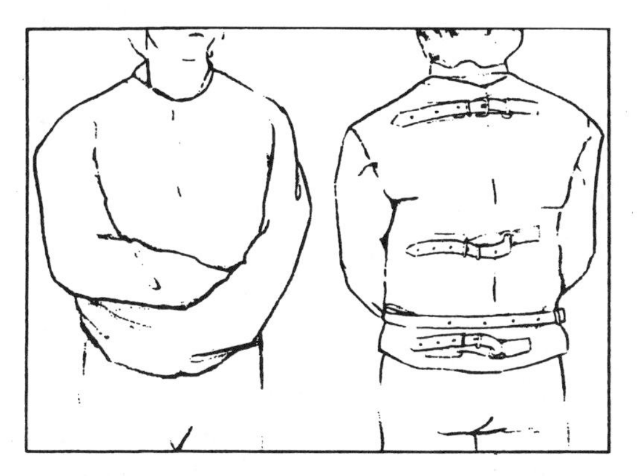

Figure 10.1 A straitjacket. (From Human Restraint Co., with permission.)

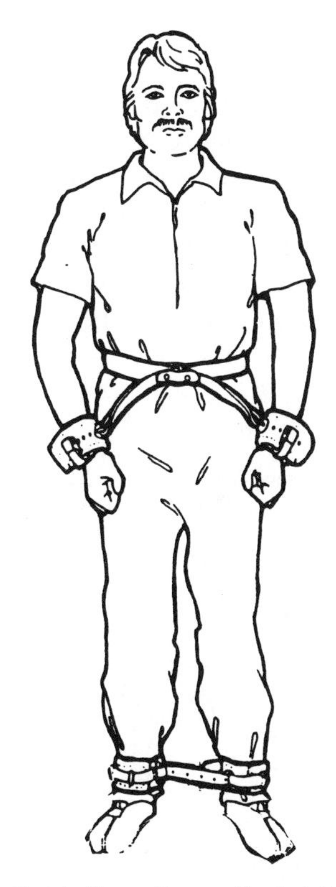

Figure 10.2 A wrist–waist restraint. (From Human Restraint Co., with permission.)

Restraints of the legs

These are basically variants on the old theme of shackles but now made of leather rather than metallic chain. They usually restrict the legs by attaching to the ankles or knees and may well have a vertical webbing attachment to a waist belt. In some cases, the arms may be fastened to the same belt, making a four-point contact.

Total body restraints

These can take the form of sheets or wet and dry packs. These are wrapped around the body of the violent person to hold him fast until he is calm. They usually require an experienced team of efficient people to operate them. Another body restraint is the 'body-bag', which is similar to a sleeping bag in which 'the patients are restrained so that they can't hurt themselves or someone else. It almost snuggles them, giving the sensation of being swaddled, giving them a greater sense of comfort' (Salvatore 1993).

Bed restraints

A number of bed restraints have been developed, including the four-point restraint. This is a bed with four straps and cuffs in the positions of hands and feet to hold the violent patient lying either prone or supine (Figs 10.3 and 10.4). Hay & Cromwell (1980) report a pipe-frame bed only a few inches high above the floor to which the frame is fixed; a thin mattress is placed upon it and four-point restraints are used. There is also the Emory cubicle bed (Williams, Morton & Patrick 1990), which is a padded frame that encompasses the bed.

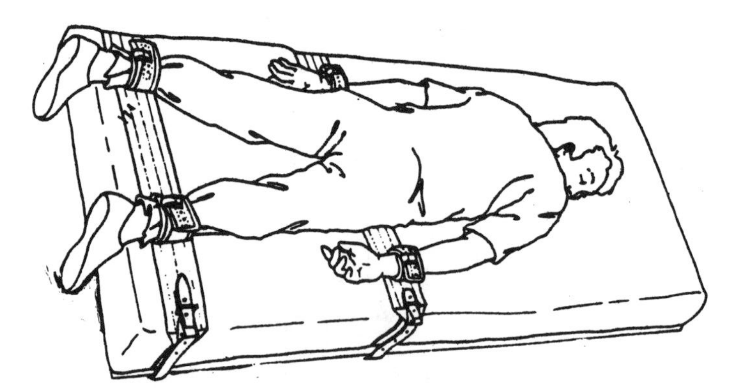

Figure 10.3 A four-point bed restraint (prone). (From Human Restraint Co., with permission.)

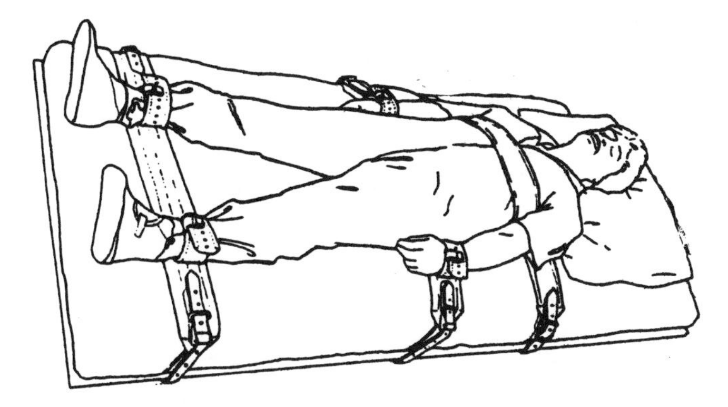

Figure 10.4 A four-point bed restraint (supine). (From Human Restraint Co., with permission.)

Mouth restraints

These are of two basic types. First are those that stop the person from biting either himself or others. Usually they are helmets of one description or another either like a fencing mask or like an American football helmet with a protective guard around the mouth. The second group consists of apparatuses that protect against spitting, which is a particularly unpleasant form of assault that can cause staff to retaliate unprofessionally with damaging consequences. A helmet with a visor has been used with good effect and in some establishments, spit shields are used when approaching disturbed aggressive individuals.

Ambulatory restraints

Ambulatory restraints in the form of preventive aggressive devices (PADs) have been pioneered by Van Rybroek et al (1987) in the USA. These devices restrict a patient's hands and/or legs but allow him to be mobile around the ward. A PAD is a belt around the waist with either long or short webbing attached to the front and ending in cuffs in which the wrists are fastened. The length of this hand webbing is adjustable and determined by the staff in response to the patient's clinical condition. At its maximum, it will allow the person to feed himself, protect himself when falling, defend himself if attacked, smoke and use the toilet whilst in the restraining device. However, assaulting another person is very difficult whilst in these restraints. They have been used successfully to shorten long-term seclusions for chronically assaultive patients (Mason 1997).

Some different ambulatory restraints are illustrated in Figure 10.5 and the differences in the freedom of arms can be noted; in (A) the wrists are restrained at the waist with no freedom of movement of the arms, in (B) the wrists are restrained at approximately 20 cm from the waist giving limited

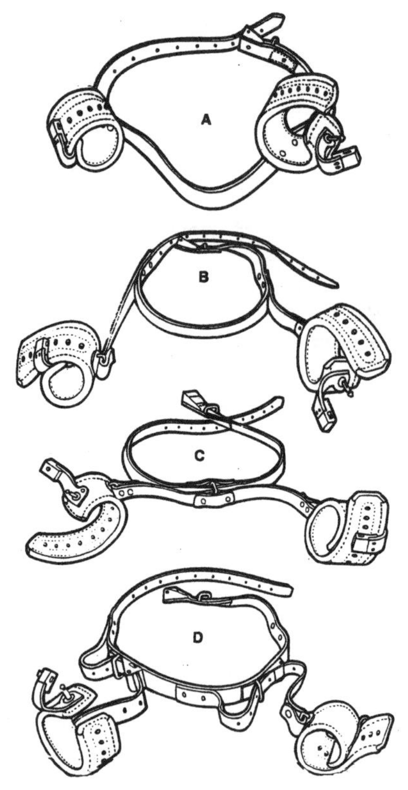

Figure 10.5 Ambulatory restraints (the Mendota PADs): **A** no freedom of arm movement; **B** limited use of arms; **C** freedom of arm movement for smoking and drinking; **D** adjustable restraint. (From Human Restraint Co., with permission.)

use of arms, in (C) the wrists are restrained at approximately 30 cm from the waist and the person can smoke or eat comfortably, and in (D) there is an adjustable restraint so wrists can be snug against the torso or given laxity of up to 30 cm, and each arm is individually adjustable.

POINTS TO REMEMBER BEFORE APPLICATION

Mechanical restraints are methods of last resort when all other interventions have been tried and failed. They should be used only in cases of extreme violence to self or others and only following agreement and with multidisciplinary involvement. The type of restraint apparatus should be determined following an extensive assessment of the patient's specific requirements. One should ensure that factors within the environment that may have caused such aggressive behaviour have been eliminated. Ensure also that the use of restraints is legitimate. Some do's and don'ts in the preparation of restraints are given in Box 10.1.

Box 10.1 Do's and don't in the preparation of restraints

Do	*Don't*
• Assess the patient thoroughly • Consult with others • Receive training in the application procedure • Ensure that all members know their role • Plan the procedure • Assess for weapons	• Take shortcuts • Ignore staff anxieties • Operate automatically without thinking • Give up on alternatives

APPLYING RESTRAINTS

The manufacturers of restraint devices should offer specific instructions on the application of their individualised apparatus. However, several principles are relevant to most types of mechanical restraints. Before applying the restraint, the patient must be under physical control if he is acting violently, as there is little point in attempting to place a cuff over a person's wrist if he is flailing and striking out. The area that will come into contact with the restraining device should be dry and free from sores or abrasions. Padding may need to be inserted between the webbing and the skin to prevent rubbing and chaffing. Ensure that the restraint is not so tight as to cause pain or restrictions in blood flow and, on the other hand, not so loose that the limb can be slipped out of the restraint. As a general rule, you should be able to slip one or two fingers between the restraint and the patient's skin. If the restraint is secured to a fixed object, make sure that if the patient attempts to move, the restraint either moves with him or does not tighten automatically.

Some do's and don'ts for the application of restraints are given in Box 10.2.

Box 10.2 Do's and don'ts in the application of restraints

Do	*Don't*
• Ensure that you are familiar with your hospital/unit policy on the use of restraints	• Secure the restraint device too tightly or too loosely
• Obtain the necessary permissions to apply the restraint before you use them	• Put restraints on wet or broken skin areas
• Ensure that you and the other members of the team are familiar with the application and use of the restraint garment	• Reprimand or degrade the patient

PROCEDURE DURING RESTRAINT USE

The patient, once in restraints, should be informed of the reasons why they have been applied, who has given authority, where he will be placed or allowed access to, and when he is likely to be released from them. There must be at least one staff member in constant attendance with the patient at all times that he is being restrained. The patient should be allowed to vent his feelings and some exploration can be undertaken as to why he became violent. Treat the patient humanely and with empathy and offer some incentive for changing his behaviour. Provide alternative courses of action for him and focus attention on him as a person. Monitor the restraint carefully ensuring that circulation is not impeded and that discomfort is not being felt. Make observations on breathing, pulse, respirations, and blood pressure as indicated. A summary of do's and don'ts for procedure whilst a patient is in restraints is given in Box 10.3.

Box 10.3 Do's and don'ts for procedure whilst a patient is in restraints

Do	*Don't*
• Change position periodically • Release restrained limb every 2 hours and stretch through range of movement • Monitor vital signs • Know how to remove the restraint in an emergency	• Forget nutrition and elimination needs • Use restraints for longer than necessary • Forget the staff will need breaks

DOCUMENTING THE USE OF RESTRAINTS

The documentation pertaining to the use of restraints is vitally important for two reasons. First, it gives a focus and a framework to ensure that the right care and management of the person is applied. Second, it is a legal safeguard if completed correctly and will offer personal, professional and organisational support in the event of litigation. An example of a documentation schedule is given in Figure 10.6.

An accompanying section for the specific observations should also be included (Fig. 10.7), which is similar to the seclusion record given in Chapter 8.

REMOVING RESTRAINTS

Restraints should be used for the shortest possible time and once the need for them has passed they should be removed immediately, but with caution. If the patient has been restrained because he is violent towards others, then it is wise to release the restraints either one at a time, if in multirestraints, or by giving increasing movement, if in PADs. At each stage, a thorough assessment of the patent's mental state should be carried out. Legs should be released before arms and you should have a second staff member standing by, at each release stage. Reinforce the patient's self-control and emphasise that full confidentiality will be maintained.

Date	Day No.	Serial No.							

Unit	Patient's name	Ward	Patient's number	Person ordering restraint Name Signature

RMO:	Primary nurse	Psychologist	Social worker

Time restraint initiated:	Time restraint terminated:

Any others involved in restraint decision
Reason for restraints Initiating/continuing
Document any PRN medication given

Name of drug	Route		Time given			Name of nurse			Form 38	Form 39	Sec 62

Type of restraint		

RELEASE REVIEW PROCESS			
Nurse in attendance	Restrained Limb Released	Time	Observations and stretching

Level of nurses in attendance	AM			PM			Nights		
	Level of nurse			Level of nurse			Level of nurse		
	1st	2nd	N/A	1st	2nd	N/A	1st	2nd	N/A
Female staff									
Male staff									
Nurse I/C signature and grade									

Figure 10.6 Documentation schedule for restraints.

<table>
<tr><td colspan="2">Name:</td><td>Day No:</td><td colspan="2">Serial No:</td><td>Date:</td></tr>
<tr><td rowspan="2">Time</td><td colspan="2" rowspan="2">Observation text at least every 15 minutes</td><td colspan="2">Cumulative times in/out of restraint</td><td rowspan="2">Name/ signature</td></tr>
<tr><td>IN</td><td>OUT</td></tr>
<tr><td>09:30</td><td colspan="2"></td><td></td><td></td><td></td></tr>
<tr><td></td><td colspan="2"></td><td></td><td></td><td></td></tr>
<tr><td></td><td colspan="2"></td><td></td><td></td><td></td></tr>
<tr><td></td><td colspan="2"></td><td></td><td></td><td></td></tr>
<tr><td colspan="6">Repeat through the 24-hour clock</td></tr>
<tr><td>Total</td><td colspan="2"></td><td></td><td></td><td></td></tr>
</table>

Figure 10.7 Observation chart for restraints.

GUIDELINES FOR THE USE OF RESTRAINTS

Organisations using restraints should have guidelines for their use; although each organisation will have its own specific requirement, there are central issues that should be addressed. The first refers to the indications for the use of restraints. Organisations should be perfectly clear about the type of behaviours that warrant mechanical restraints, from self-harming, to someone violently assaulting others. The second is concerned with the legal orders for the use of restraints. Although the multidisciplinary team should be involved in the overall debate regarding the use of restraints, the responsible medical officer (RMO) is ultimately charged with the legal responsibility and his signature is required before restraints are used. Thirdly, clinical assessments should be made, not only of the requirements for mechanical restraints, but of the risks to the patient. For example, it is important to evaluate the vulnerability of the restrained patient to, say, attack from others or falling whilst in restraints. Fourthly, the observations made during periods of restraint should be accounted for in the policy formulation and, like seclusion, a written observation should be made every 15 minutes; unlike seclusion, however, a nurse should be in constant attendance whilst the patient is being restrained. Fifthly, the release procedure should be addressed in the guidelines and include releases and stretching every 2 hours. Finally, the documentation should be clearly established and its completion emphasised. This should include restraint documentation as well as the patient's record.

Some guidelines for mechanical restraint are shown in Box 10.4.

Box 10.4 Some guidelines for mechanical restraint

1. Indications for use	(a) For use to protect the patient from self-harm (b) To prevent the patient from assaulting others
2. Legal requirements	(a) Multidisciplinary involvement (b) RMO's signature (c) Patient advocacy/relative (d) Patient agreement
3. Clinical assessments	(a) Patient's mental state (b) Risks to the patient (c) Need for restraints
4. Observations	(a) Nurse in constant attendance (b) Written record every 15 minutes (c) Release limb from restraint every 2 hours (d) Stretch limb through range of movement (e) Monitor vital signs (f) Observe blood flow (g) Observe the restraint is not rubbing
5. Release procedure	(a) Limit on time in restraint (b) Behaviours required before release (c) Two-hourly release procedure (d) Terminating restraints
6. Documentation	(a) Restraint documentation (b) Patient's record (c) Day report

ADVANTAGES AND DISADVANTAGES OF MECHANICAL RESTRAINT

The advantages and disadvantages of mechanical restraints are first and foremost concerned with the ethical implications for their use. When seen in relation to the behaviour that their use is attempting to prevent (i.e. self-injury or serious harm to others), then mechanical restraints are less harmful than those behaviours themselves. Therefore, they can be viewed as morally appropriate. However, when seen in relation to other modes of preventing such violence (e.g. chemical control) they appear more restrictive. Therefore, they can also be viewed as morally unjustified. Mental health workers having to debate these issues are faced with difficult choices about the preferred mode of intervention for those patients who are chronically assaultive. Whereas some believe that long periods of seclusion are less distasteful than mechanical restraints, others have argued that chemical control is more humane. However, with modern mechanical restraints allowing some degree of ambulation whilst restricting the possibilities of assault, there are also those who believe that such devices are better than either chemical control or seclusion (Stolley et al 1993).

Advantages

The advantages of the use of mechanical restraint include the fact that the patient is not left alone and always has a nurse in constant attendance. This allows for interaction and the communication of positive feedback, which is not so readily achievable, either with seclusion, or when someone is tranquillised through medication. Mechanical restraint allows the person to vent his anger but keeps him safe from damaging others or property. Modern restraints allow the person to feed, smoke and toilet independently and give a degree of autonomy, which chemical control and seclusion take away. Mechanical restraint is a specialised procedure calling for skilled nursing and cumulative experience. Such specialist skills require training, practice and updating and should be part of in-service development. The application of restraints, and the care and management of people in them, therefore requires specialist nurses. This gives the procedure a depth and scope that eliminates the use of restraints for convenience purposes in which the patient is forgotten. A skilled nurse will bring to the procedure, all the interactive approaches that mental health nursing incorporates and will give the application of mechanical restraints a quality that otherwise would be reduced. Another advantage of mechanical restraint is the multidisciplinary approach that accompanies it. Whereas the use of medication and seclusion rooms can tend to leave the patient isolated and marginalised, once the crisis is under control, the use of mechanical restraint is high profile and needs constant nursing input as well as multidisciplinary reviews.

Disadvantages

There are, of course, disadvantages to the use of mechanical restraint; these range from mild to severe, as there are a number of fatalities attributed to its use. The main area of disadvantage concerns the patient being neglected. If the restraints are used because the patient's behaviour is inconvenient, troublesome or consuming too much nursing time, then it is being used illegitimately and is inviting problems. The emphasis must always be on a specialist nurse in constant attendance to a patient who is being mechanically restrained. There are a number of corollaries to this neglect, which include patients suffering from sensory deprivation due to protracted times spent in restraints. If limbs are fixed for long periods, the patient can suffer from a distorted body image and, as can be imagined, the practice would also contribute to an unhealthy dependence on nursing staff and form the basis of inappropriate regressed behaviours. Prolonged immobilisation can also cause biophysiological dysfunctions such as loss of appetite, dehydration, skin breakdown and hypoxia (Archea et al 1993). Continued restraints for long periods can also cause a loss of interest in exercise and a decrease in muscle mass. There are also reports of 'incontinence, loss of the ability to walk, depression, fear, panic and accentuation of cognitive impairment occur frequently. Elimination problems and cardiac stress have also been observed' (Archea et al 1993, p. 6). Clearly, these are serious disadvantages to the use of mechanical restraints and can be seen as a result of bad nursing practice of patients in such apparatuses.

An area of especial disadvantage in the use of mechanical restraint is concerned with inappropriate use for specified target behaviours. When used for extremes of violence, they appear to be more effective in reducing such aggression. However, if the person is left in restraint for longer than is necessary, or placed in restraints when compliant, then patients can become antagonistic to the restraint as well as to those applying them. They can become agitated and more aggressive, both verbally and physically.

Deaths have also been reported for patients who have been mechanically restrained. Robinson, Sucholeiki & Schocken (1993) reported a case of an elderly man who had resisted mechanical restraints and suddenly died. The post mortem claimed that he had died as a result of what was established as a plausible link between restraint, psychological stress and sudden death. Miles (1993) also gave an account of an elderly lady who had died in a similar manner. The lady had senile dementia and was confused by the restraint. She had escaped from the jacket restraint and was 'raving, biting, kicking and scratching' (Miles 1993, p. 1013). She was described as 'working on the restraints' and suddenly died. Weick (1992) claimed that more than 50 deaths were attributed to mechanical restraints between 1984 and 1992. The age range of those who had died was between 10 and 90 years, which shows the extent of its use in the USA. The main reasons why patients had died were because of incorrect usage of restraint, the patient resisting, the patient not being monitored, the patient not being regularly freed and the wrong choice of restraint apparatus.

CONCLUSIONS

In this chapter we have seen that the use of mechanical restraints for violent persons has become much refined in recent years. This refinement takes the form of customised restraints developed for specific individuals with distinctively aggressive traits. Modern-day restraints allow for greater flexibility in the range of movement and ambulation whilst affording some control over assaultive behaviour. They are often made of leather or strong webbing and have soft padding to protect against chaffing or rubbing. Mechanical restraints require specialised nurses, trained and experienced in the practice, to apply and monitor patients who are thus restrained.

There are serious concerns regarding the use of mechanical restraint, as there are with other types of interventions, for extremely violent persons;

these have ethical, legal, organisational and professional dimensions. Ethically, we need to address issues of liberty, reasonableness and the least restrictive alternative. Legal concerns should be dealt with by the involvement of multidisciplinary teams, responsible medical officer, the patient, patient's advocates, patient's relatives and legal representatives where necessary. Documentation is vitally important in these matters, both to safeguard good practice and to protect against litigation. Health organisations are charged with providing treatment and management of patients in environments that are both healthy and safe for its workers. Professional issues are concerned with the provision of high-quality patient care in a manner that operates in the best interests of the patient. Mechanical restraint produces visual images that prick consciences and are unpleasant in ideal worlds. It is this visual imagery that allows for more invisible practices to become more professionally acceptable.

Note

Special thanks are extended to the Humane Restraint Co. Inc., 912 Bethel Circle, Waunakee, Wisconsin 53597, USA, who gave kind permission to reproduce their drawings in Figures 10.1–10.5.

11

Chemical control

KEY POINTS

1. The use of drugs is the preferred option among the patients surveyed.
2. Forced medication is strongly objected to by patients.
3. Effective use of PRN medication can reduce the need for emergency administration.
4. Emergency use of medication needs careful planning.
5. There are differing approaches to the use of emergency medication.

INTRODUCTION

In Chapter 10, we discussed the role of mechanical restraints in the management of violence and aggression, and the fact that no matter how these forms of restraints are presented, the image that remains is one of harsh barbarity. With medication used as a form of restraint, the problems of image are subtly different. We have deliberately placed this chapter on medication immediately after that on mechanical restraint and have used the title of 'chemical control' to maintain as blunt an image as possible. The rationale for this is that in the phase of assault, management is often harsh, unpleasant and 'not pretty' (Maier & Van Rybroek 1990). Furthermore, in dealing with the extremes of violence, it is the fact that the major concerns involve the integrity of the human body, in terms both of the personal injuries that can be sustained by staff and patients, and also of the necessity to stop the attacker, and this usually involves breaching the integrity of his body. The types of control used to restrain the assaultive person must, by necessity, have a close relationship to the body. In the throes of combat, the use of isolation techniques secludes the person alone, thus protecting others, and allows the combatant some degree of movement around the room or area. Thus the controlling forces of the walls and locked doors are at some distance from the body or the person directly. With the use of physical and mechanical restraints, the controlling forces are either the personnel holding the attacker or the mechanisms limiting his movement; even with ambulatory restraints they are in contact with the body, and one can imagine the forces of control lying so close to the human body as to follow its contours, as close as a straitjacket, immobilising the person completely. With medication, the forces of control slip beneath the external parameters of the body and lie within, coursing through the veins, synapses and cells, deep inside the body.

Whereas seclusion rooms, mechanical apparatuses and staff physically holding the combatant are highly visible entities, chemicals to some degree lie hidden within the body. The former types of control produce images that disturb the senses more so than do drugs administered to the patient. Although we see their side-effects, which can be most unpleasant and sometimes dangerous, the accompanying images are misinterpreted as peaceful sleep or manifestations of the patient's clinical state, rather than the drugs themselves. It appears to us that this invisibility is one main reason why, in the debate concerning the ethical implications of using the various forms of restraint, the use of drugs tends to be more acceptable than that of the other forms of control. In a study of patient choice regarding the use of seclusion, restraints and the use of either benzodiazepines or neuroleptics, patients preferred medication (64%) to either seclusion or restraints (36%). However, through rank ordering, it became clear that in terms of strength of objection, many patients were more opposed to the forced medication than to other forms of restraint (Sheline & Nelson 1993). Another reason for the preferred choice of medication may possibly be related to the extent to which drug companies invest in the development of medications through research and marketing. Whatever the reasons for the use of chemicals in the control of violence and aggression, most mental health centres, but by no means all, do use drugs to one degree or another in the management of these behaviours.

THERAPEUTIC USE OF DRUGS

We have pointed out in several areas of this book that we are predominantly concerned with the management of violence and aggression in the crisis stage, in which control of the combatant person is of paramount importance. Notwithstanding this, we appreciate that this phase is not clearly delineated with distinct boundaries between the build-up or the calm-down and that, as we noted in Chapter 3, the transition to and from the phase of combat differs according to the individual, the circumstance and the context. Therefore, before concentrating on the use of chemicals in the crisis of combat, we would like to briefly mention the extended use of medication in the longer-term therapeutic approach to the management of violence.

Neuroleptics

The therapeutic use of medication falls roughly into four main groups. The first are what are known as neuroleptics. These are used mainly for the schizophrenias, manias and in some cases, for organic disorders that are associated with delusional beliefs with tendencies towards violence. They can also be used for agitated depression and toxic delirium; however, in these conditions they are used for a shorter term. The neuroleptics tranquillise patients without causing paradoxical excitement and are thought to act by interfering with the transmission of dopamine by blocking receptors. There are four main types. First are those that cause a pronounced sedative effect with moderate side-effects, for example, chlorpromazine, methotrimeprazine and promazine. The second have a lesser sedating effect but also fewer side-effects, for example, thioridazine, pericyazine and pipothiazine. The third category is less sedating but has more pronounced side-effects and includes fluphenazine, prochlorperazine and trifluoperazine. Finally, there are drugs that have a combination of reactions in various degrees; these include droperidol, haloperidol, pimozide, flupenthixol and clozapine. Like all drugs, the neuroleptics have certain side-effects. These include extrapyramidal symptoms of the Parkinsonian type, for instance dystonia, akathisia and tardive dyskinesia. Side-effects also include hypotension, disturbances of temperature regulation and the rare, but potentially fatal, neuroleptic malignancy syndrome (NMS).

Beta blockers

The second group of drugs used in the therapeutic management of violence and aggression is the beta blockers. These drugs have been used with aggressive patients with organic brain diseases and impairments that are secondary to trauma. They have also been successfully used in some mental impairment states including dementia, Huntington's chorea and Korsakoff's psychosis. The main drug of choice is propanolol; however, there are many conditions in which this drug should not be used.

Anticonvulsants

The third group of drugs is the anticonvulsants, which have been used effectively in managing aggression in schizophrenic patients with or without electroencephalogram abnormalities, and also in personality-disordered patients with or without brain damage. Again, there are a number of side-effects, some of which are serious but rare. The main drugs used are carbamazepine and sodium valproate.

Lithium

The final group of drugs used for violence comprises lithium. This medication is mainly used for the management of bipolar affective disorder; however, it has also been used effectively for violent patients with 'organic brain syndrome, aggressive schizophrenics, non-psychotics, aggressive prisoners, delinquents, and children with conduct disorders and attention deficit' (Tardiff 1992, p. 562).

This is of course, a brief overview of the therapeutic long-term approach to the chemical treatment of violence and aggression. These drugs are mentioned merely to reflect that some decisions made at the time of the crisis about which drugs are given to disturbed individuals can have ramifications for the longer-term management.

THE USE OF PRN MEDICATION

In the chemical management of a violent episode, the use of PRN is often the first mode of intervention. PRN medication is the use of a prescribed drug given to the patient as needed rather than at predetermined times. 'As needed', therefore, suggests that there is a changing clinical picture, altering dynamically through the course of time, in response to a multifaceted reticulate of influences. It also connotes that an ongoing assessment is being conducted of the extent to which the conditions are changing in relation to the need for the medication to be taken, in short, that there is an evaluation of how much the 'as needed' is needed.

Assessment dimensions

The PRN assessment has two dimensions. These are first, an assessment undertaken by the person who is going to receive the medication, who then approaches staff and requests the PRN. The second dimension involves an assessment undertaken by others, who then either persuade the person that they should take the medication or force them to take it within legal and professional parameters.

These assessments are, in fact, qualitatively different and involve diverse perspectives depending upon who is performing the assessment (i.e. the person receiving the drug or the person who will administer it). In the former case, where the person undertaking the assessment will be the one to ingest it, he will be experiencing internal phenomena that underline his evaluation of their need. These may include 'positive' experiences that appear real to the patient such as hallucinations, delusions, tenseness, worry, agitation and so on. Or, alternatively, it may well be 'negative' experiences of wishing to satisfy an addiction, to induce an alternative conscious state through the use of PRN drugs, to seek attention, or to falsely portray an image of disturbed behaviour for secondary gains. The important point is that the person experiences *something* that directly precipitates a request for medication. A second consequence of this form of assessment is that it allows for patients who consider that they do not need PRN medication but who may well be suffering from considerable disturbance. This brings us into the domain of the second dimension of assessment: assessment by others who are not going to receive the medication themselves but who may experience consequences of their decision.

In assessing that another person may need PRN medication, one is making value judgements about another person's physical and psychological state and adjudging that the intervention will, in effect, help the patient maintain a state of equilibrium. This in turn, draws upon assumptions concerning the relationship between (a) perceived signs and symptoms, (b) consequences of non-PRN use and (c) the possibility of the intervention being effective if applied. Furthermore, although the administration of PRN will have some effect on the patient, this may not be the anticipated or desired effect. Additionally, we need to be aware of the motivations of clinicians administering PRN and to ensure that these are for the best interests of the patient and the well-being of others, and not merely the desire for peace and quiet.

It may also well be that administering PRN drugs may mask the development of unwanted side-effects of other prescribed medication. Alternatively, it may mask a worsening condition; for example, administering a sedating neuroleptic to an apparently increasingly disturbed psychotic person who is engaging in facial grimacing could suppress signs of developing tardive dyskinesia. Therefore, what becomes evident in this rather long preamble to the assessment for the administration of PRN is that the matter is far more complicated than merely requesting the patient to take some medication.

Administration considerations

In the vast majority of cases, it is the nurse who initiates the administration of PRN (McLaren, Browne & Taylor 1990), the reasons for this initiative being many and varied (Fishel et al 1994). In practical terms, the signs and symptoms that give rise to the decision to give PRN medication can range from the obviously important to the apparently insignificant. The crucial element in assessing for PRN administration is the extent to which the indications observed have been known to lead, in the past, to behaviour or mental states that are undesirable or dangerous. For example, if a patient is known to resort to violence following the painting of bizarre signs on his face, it may be appropriate to offer PRN medication as soon as this is manifested in an attempt to prevent violence occurring. However, the documented rationale for the administration of PRN may be 'to prevent aggression' rather than because he was 'painting his face'.

The main reasons for PRN use are summarised in Table 11.1.

Once the decision to administer PRN is taken, it should be done persuasively and with the interests of the patient foremost. Knowledge of the patient is crucial for achieving good results in giving PRN and there are several approaches that can be adopted depending upon the nature of the staff–patient relationship and the experience in dealing with specific individuals:

1. Nonchalant approach – in this, the patient is approached in an easy manner, light heartedly, with a brief explanation given of what is going on, and then the medication offered without fuss.
2. 'Your best interests' approach – this calls for contact with the patient who is then reasoned with; the central message is that 'this is in your best interests'.
3. 'For the sake of others' approach – in this, the central message is that there is a deterioration in the patient's mental state and in the past this has led to others getting hurt.

Table 11.1 Main reasons for use of PRN

Reason for PRN	Main reference source
Agitation	Craven, Voore & Voineskos 1987
Relief of distress	McLaren, Browne & Taylor 1990
Prevention of aggression	McLaren, Browne & Taylor 1990
Containment of aggression	McLaren, Browne & Taylor 1990
Hostility	Mason & DeWolfe 1974
Overactivity	Mason & DeWolfe 1974
Assaultiveness	Mason & DeWolfe 1974
Hallucinations	Mason & DeWolfe 1974
Destructiveness	Mason & DeWolfe 1974
Agitation	Fishel et al 1994
Insomnia	Fishel et al 1994

4. Straight-talking approach – in this, the patient is approached in a friendly but firm manner and the facts of the situation are briefly explained, slowly and honestly, with the consequences outlined in a professional way.

The situational differences of these approaches are vast and decisions should be taken as to whether it is best to approach the patient directly, manoeuvre the patient into an isolated position, or request a private meeting with him in a quiet part of the unit.

Care and planning should be undertaken to cover all eventualities and both you and the team should be aware of their responses should the patient:

- decline the medication
- refuse in an aggressive manner
- throw the medication away
- become verbally abusive
- run away
- attack.

Procedure following administration

Following successful administration of the medication, there are a number of observations and actions to be undertaken. First, PRN medication has a favourable outcome when successfully administered. Observe the patient for signs of:

1. increasing/decreasing signs of the original disturbed behaviour (i.e. the rationale for deciding on PRN in the first instance)
2. increasing/decreasing signs of related psychopathology (e.g. anxiety, agitation, hostility, etc.)
3. the onset of side-effects
4. any other response from the patient.

Unfortunately, sometimes PRN is not prescribed, fails to be offered when it is, or is not successfully administered, and then an emergency situation develops that calls for swift intervention of chemical control.

EMERGENCY ADMINISTRATION

Administering medication in an emergency situation is a procedure that is fraught with many dangers and can have serious ramifications in terms of the biopsychological consequences for the patient, as well as ethical, legal and professional concerns for those administering the drug. Clearly, the administration by health professionals of drugs in emergency situations is highly likely to be in contrived circumstances in a set procedure carried out in health care settings under the appropriate legislation and within the guidelines of independent authority policies and procedures. The emergency situation will usually, but not exclusively, call for the forced administration of medication intramuscularly or intravenously; although trained nursing staff may operate the former, in the latter case, a medical staff member should undertake this procedure. Staff members need to be very clear about the legal considerations, which in the UK are governed by the Mental Health Act (1983), part IV on consent to treatment. The relevant sections are sections 57 and 58, which pertain to treatment requiring consent or a second opinion, section 60, which is the withdrawal of consent, and section 62, on the need for urgent treatment. Other countries have their respective legislation, while practice in the USA is restricted by individual state laws. The important point is that most countries who accept this form of chemical restraint in the welfare of disturbed individuals, do so, under the auspices of a legislative framework.

There is also a need to appreciate that, although most psychiatric patients, who have been surveyed prefer the use of medication in the emergency situation, there was a strong indication that this is when it is taken orally or acceded to voluntarily (Fishel et al 1994). When it is a question of having the medication forced into a patient who is struggling against it, there is a clear rejection of this form of restraint. Whereas a person can be freed from a seclusion room or have physical restraints removed, once injected, the medication must run its course. To have a drug within one's body against one's will and holding some control over one's actions, with possibly strange side-effects such as hypersalivation, must surely be a personally degrading and disturbingly worrying situation (Deschamp 1994). This may have profound effects for any form of therapeutic nurse–patient relationship.

However, once the legal, ethical and professional issues have been resolved and the decision is made that this form of chemical control is deemed appropriate, then some practical concerns also need to be addressed. We will focus in the next section on the emergency administration of the intramuscular injection of a person who is resisting the procedure, while accepting that at varying stages of the exercise, the patient should be requested to comply.

ASSESSMENT PROCEDURE

Prior to any action, an assessment should be carried out, and clearly, the longer one appraises this, the more thorough it can be. However, even in those moments of crisis when a situation has occurred, apparently spontaneously, some form of assessment should be conducted. It is helpful to establish an assessment strategy that incorporates a number of areas, which then can be drawn upon to provide an overall evaluation and plan. The plan should address the following six areas:

1. Assessment – assess as much as you can in the time given to you.
2. Ensure safety – for the patient, staff and others who are likely to become involved.
3. Communication – keep talking and reassuring the patient that he will be taken care of.
4. Continuity of care – provision must be made for continuity of care following a satisfactory resolution to the crisis.
5. Medication – ensure that the medication given is based on the most appropriate assessment and is prescribed correctly.
6. Legal concerns – ensure that your practice complies to legal requirements (i.e. minimum force required in the least restrictive manner).

The first assessment is an evaluation of the patient, which should include both internal and external factors (Box 11.1).

Box 11.1 Internal and external assessment factors

Internal	*External*
Apparent psychopathology, hallucinations, delusions	Sequence of events
Level of control, muscle tension, posturing, uncooperativeness, excitement, staring	Precipitating events
Extent of anxiety, agitation	Environmental factors
Size, weight and strength of patient	Involvement of others, family, friends, peers, staff
Extent of threatening behaviour, including specific target	Specificity of target
Levels of distress	Interpersonal relations, family, friends, peers, staff
Previous history	Accessibility to weapons
Ingestion of substances	Availability of support team
	Peer involvement

Internal factors

Internal factors are those that involve the patient's mental state or behaviour. The assessment of the mental state should incorporate the establishment of a baseline from which future evaluations can be assessed. They include whether the patient is experiencing hallucinations, with an indication of whether he is resisting or responding to this experience. A note should be made of the extent of any delusional activity to which a response may provoke an attack. The levels of anxiety, agitation, muscle tension and excitement should be observed and verbal attempts should be undertaken to calm the situation where appropriate.

Behavioural indicators will also include the level of internal control, or otherwise, that the patient is achieving, and whether he is posturing, staring at a specific target, threatening a specific action, or exhibiting generalised hostility, and the levels of distress that are manifested. Other factors to be considered are the size, weight and strength of the patient to ensure enough support is available to overcome him if necessary, in the least restrictive manner and with the minimum force required. Previous knowledge of the patient in these scenarios should be reviewed, and the extent to which these actions led to certain consequences. It is worth noting here that if a particular previous action by staff has successfully resolved the situation, then it may be worth attempting this again. Similarly, if a particular action was unsuccessful previously, then avoid attempting it again in this situation unless it has been modified. Also assess whether the patient is likely to have ingested substances that may have contributed to his current state; it is wise to remember that he may well be in an extremely disinhibited state if this is the case.

External factors

External factors are those influences on the patient emanating from the environment, or are frustrations to his actions. They may include restrictions on his movements, lack of immediate gratification of his wishes, having to wait for something, or not being able to access something he desires. There should also be an assessment of the sequence of events that led to this situation developing, as the precipitant cause may continue to influence him negatively and its removal, if possible, could ease the situation. For instance, the patient may be experiencing environment excesses such as loud noise, heat or cold, or could possibly be finding the intensity of relationships with family, friends, peers or staff members to be excessive. One also needs to assess his availability to any threatened or intended victims, who should be removed for their protection and in the hope of defusing the situation. Assessment should also be undertaken in relation to the patient's availability to arm himself with weapons. Finally, one should assess the number, skills and experience of the support team, as well as the possible response from the patient's peers who may join in the struggle in his 'defence'.

The above is not an exhaustive list of factors to be assessed but provides a general framework on which many other indicators could be mapped in the overall evaluation. Many situations, and individuals, have unique aspects that should be incorporated in the assessment and all should contribute to establishing a plan and the construction of baselines for future assessments.

PLANNING AND PREPARATION

Planning is a vitally important aspect of any procedure and this is especially the case when considering chemical control of the violent patient. Often the lack of time does not allow for detailed and intricate organisation of the procedure, especially when working in acute areas since the situations that are faced often require a swift response. However, in areas where emergency situations are relatively common, general planning of the procedure for administering emergency medication should be undertaken. This should include such aspects as ensuring access to emergency provisions, (e.g. airways, resuscitation equipment, intravenous infusions, cut-down sets and emergency drugs). An area of the unit should be designated and familiar to all staff members and they should be aware that this is where the emergency administration of drugs will take place.

Staff preparation

The role of particular staff members in the event of an emergency occurring should be understood and there should be periodic rehearsals of emergencies. The psychiatric crisis is not too dissimilar to the situation of cardiac arrest in which equipment is on stand-by and members of the 'crash' team know their specific role and receive training in the procedure. Therefore, if one adopts this principle of planning, the potential chaos of psychiatric emergencies can be minimised.

Unfortunately, in one sense each emergency situation is unique and needs to be responded to as events occur. Therefore, experience and typification are of paramount importance. Experience brings a degree of foresight and a certain knowledge of possible outcomes, and typification allows us to assess situations relative to previous experiences and their resolution (see Chapter 14). These indicators are influential in the planning stage. It is suggested that the following should be reviewed:

1. ensure that staff members understand their role
2. ensure that the staff have the capacity to fulfil their role
3. ensure baselines are recorded where possible
4. keep calm
5. act decisively.

Preparation of area

The area used for the administration of medicine should be prepared, ensuring that obstacles are removed and any items that could be used as a weapon are secured. If restraints are being used, then these should be prepared. The medication should be made ready, ensuring that both oral and intramuscular preparations are available where possible. In most circumstances where planning and time allow, medical staff should be involved in the process and be prepared for the eventuality of medical emergencies.

Restraint use

Depending upon the situation, the violently struggling patient may need to be restrained. If appropriate ask him to comply with your requests, or otherwise, use the most suitable method of restraint as outlined in chapters 9 and 10. If the seclusion room is to be used for administering the injection, then transfer the patient to this facility and lie the patient face down whilst maintaining control of him. Remove any items of security and any clothing needed to access the injection site. If mechanical restraints are to be used then these should be applied. If not, the patient should be held firmly whilst the injection is given. Spit shields should be used if the person is engaging in spitting behaviour.

ADMINISTERING THE DRUGS

The patient should always be offered the medication orally if possible as this provides some degree of choice and control for him. If he refuses, or the situation is such that the quicker action of intramuscular injection is required for safety reasons, then this should be undertaken. There are differing approaches to chemical control of the violent patient depending upon the type of drugs used and the overall approach to the management of the patient.

Rapid sedation

Where it is decided that the patient requires sedating, possibly because of acute excitement and aggressively disturbed behaviour, but where long-term chemical management is not considered appropriate, the benzodiazepines are often the drugs of preference. Lorazepam, either alone or in combination with other drugs, is a popular choice. Advocates of this drug have argued that as the target symptoms requiring rapid sedation are non-specific (i.e. tension, excitement and anxiety) and accompanied by varying degrees of aggression, lorazepam sedates the patient well without the risks of extrapyramidal symptoms or NMS (p. 196) (Dubin & Feld 1989). In reviewing the literature, Dubin & Feld (1989) reported that doses ranged from 2–4 mg i.m. up to 120 mg in 24 hours with the 'maximum single dose as 30 mg orally, 16 mg i.m. and 80 mg i.v. over 40 minutes' (p. 317). However, there is little consensus regarding single dosage, the time intervals between doses and the ceiling dose, which places the responsibility for deciding this on the prescribing doctor.

Other drugs used for rapid sedation include midazolam, which is generally used as a preanaesthetic (Mendoza, Djenderedjian & Adams 1987), and droperidol, an analogue of haloperidol, which has been used in assaultive and severely agitated patients (Resnick & Burton 1984).

Droperidol has no antipsychotic action but has good sedating qualities. Barbiturates, such as sodium amytal, have also been used but without literature to support this. The last group of drugs tend to produce many side-effects and have problems of withdrawal.

Rapid neuroleptisation

Rapid neuroleptisation, also called psychotolysis, is a procedure used for severely disturbed individuals where antipsychotic medication is administered rapidly, in the first instance to control the patient, and then to continue the medication to control the symptoms. Observations of pulse, blood pressure, temperature and respiration should be taken prior to the administration of neuroleptics. Clearly, with violently struggling patients, this is not achievable, nor would such measurements be particularly accurate as a baseline measure. However, once the medication has been administered and the patient is becoming more controlled, then vital signs should be taken. As the aggression subsides, these observations should be undertaken at approximately 15 minute intervals since hypotension can occur as a side-effect of neuroleptisation.

The main drug of choice is haloperidol, a butyrophenone, which is effective in controlling severely disturbed and agitated patients and suppressing psychotic symptoms. It is a drug considered to be relatively free from side-effects and can cause a reduction in violence within 20 minutes of being administered by intramuscular injection. Droperidol, as mentioned above, is an analogue of haloperidol that is faster acting and with good sedating qualities. Droperidol can begin to reduce violent tendencies within 5 minutes of injection but it does need an antipsychotic combination drug to counteract the psychosis. Extrapyramidal side-effects have been observed with both haloperidol and droperidol, the main responses being dystonias and tremors. There have also been reports of euphoria, headaches, confusion and vertigo (Deschamp 1994).

These drugs may be prescribed every 30 minutes until the patient calms down and the correct titration is achieved. In the literature, it has been reported that most disturbed patients come under control after 6 to 10 hours of rapid neuroleptisation with the majority becoming calm a lot sooner (Piotrowski 1979). At this stage, the route of administration can usually be switched to oral preparations. A number of formulas have been used for converting from intramuscular to oral routes. For example, some adopt a doubling formula, for example 40 mg i.m. would convert to 80 mg orally in divided doses with the main dose given at night. Others have used an 80% conversion ratio with good effect. Again, some physicians convert from intramuscular to oral administration on the same day, whilst others prefer to convert to oral only on the following day after intramuscular injections have controlled the patient. Once converted to oral administration, the drug is maintained for a period of time depending upon the clinical status of the patient; then the dosage is tapered down until a therapeutic balance is achieved.

Side-effects

Although we have mentioned the side-effects that can occur with chemical control throughout the chapter, here, we would like to mention briefly some aspects of side-effects and their management that is specifically related to the drugs used in neuroleptisation. Most drugs that are administered have a number of effects on the body; for example, the common drug aspirin, which is usually taken as an analgesic for headaches, also produces gastrointestinal irritation and increases bleeding time because of its antiplatelet action, amongst many other things. The former side-effect may well be unwanted but the latter one may be desirable as it may be used for prophylaxis in cerebrovascular disease or myocardial infarction. There is a need to balance risks and requirements and decide about the acceptability of consequences for taking or not taking certain medicine, and this is as much the case for aspirin as it is for neuroleptics.

Dystonia

The main group of side-effects from sedatives and neuroleptics are the extrapyramidal symptoms, the most common being dystonia. A dystonic reaction comprises a sudden turning and twisting caused by sustained muscular contractions, which is often misdiagnosed as some form of hysterical conversion. As facial muscles are also affected, there can be grimacing with the eyes being pulled upwards (occulogyric crisis). A second common side-effect is akathisia, literally meaning an inability to sit still, with resultant pacing, restlessness, tenseness and irritability. The treatment for both these conditions is usually the administration of benztropine (Cogentin) or benzhexol (Artane), which are anti-Parkinsonian drugs. Extrapyramidal symptoms are usually quite mild and reversible although unpleasant until counteracted.

Neuroleptic malignancy syndrome (NMS)

Another side-effect of the neuroleptics is of greater concern. This is NMS, which is a serious reaction involving autonomic instability with hyperthermia, hypertension and rigidity as common features. Fortunately, it occurs only in approximately 1% of cases and with growing knowledge of factors that place patients at risk for NMS, some avoidance of this side-effect is achievable. These include: 'young, chronic, male patients who are dehydrated, malnourished, and placed in poorly ventilated seclusion rooms or in restraints' (Dubin & Feld 1989; p. 316). This potentially fatal condition requires discontinuation of drug therapy as there is no established treatment, although bromocriptine and dantrolene have been used. Following discontinuance of drug therapy, the condition can last for approximately 5–10 days, and longer, if depot injections have been used.

DOCUMENTATION

The documentation pertaining to the administration of emergency medication is vitally important not only because it is a legal requirement but also because, in emergency situations, drugs are often prescribed verbally. In these circumstances, there will be specific requirements depending on individual authority/hospital policies. In some cases, verbal instructions regarding medications are not permitted, whilst in others, two qualified nurses must verify the verbal prescription. Depending upon specific policy requirements, ensure that the documentation is completed as it may be important at a later date in legal proceedings, in the event of an inquest, inquiry or litigation. Figure 11.1 is a general guideline of factors that should be recorded.

ADVANTAGES AND DISADVANTAGES OF DRUG USE

The advantages and disadvantages of using drugs for the control and management of the violent patient in the emergency situation are, again, a question of personal perspectives (Box 11.2).

Advantages

Advantages may include the rapid control of disturbed behaviour with or without violence and aggression, which may have been raging for some considerable time and may have impacted on family, friends or other patients. Such interventions, therefore, bring relief not only to the patient, but also to many others. The relief of distressing symptoms can in itself be viewed as an advantage as it helps the patient orientate himself and reintegrates him into society. Coping mechanisms are re-established and cognitive functioning becomes improved. Swift intervention in a psychiatric crisis with the use of medication may signal to the patient that staff are attempting to help him in this difficult time. This may aid in establishing a more trusting relationship formation and show family and friends that help is being given that will contribute overall towards a therapeutic atmosphere. Engaging the patient's illness can establish rapport with all concerned and reassure everyone that the person's condition is not permanent. In cases of acute psychiatric decompensation, in which there is increased anxiety over the loss of

Name		D.O.B.				Baselines			
Weight		Allergies				B/P	T	P	R
Drug	Drug	Dose	Route	Freq.	Signature				
1/4/97	Haloperidol	20mg	I.M.	Stat					
1/4/97	Artane	2mg	O.	PRN					

State of Consciousness

Rousable 1. Needs physical prompting 2. Unresponsive 3.

Date	Time	Drug	Scale	Other observations

Further comments and special instructions

Signature

Figure 11.1 Documentation for emergency medication.

Box 11.2 Advantages and disadvantages of chemical control

Advantages	*Disadvantages*
Rapid control of disturbed behaviour	Many side-effects of various drugs used
Brings relief of symptoms for patient and others	Damage to injection site
Helps the patient orientate himself	Forced medication is dehumanising
Coping mechanisms are improved	
Helps form trusting relationship	
Establishes rapport with all concerned	
Shows condition is not permanent	
Patient not abandoned	
Can lead to day case treatment	

control over one's own impulses, demonstrating to the patient that he was not abandoned and that re-establishing control was prompt, aids a fuller recovery. Other advantages include the quick transfer to day-patient treatment where family and friends take a more active role in treatment, which allows daily contact with the patient and provides an opportunity for assisting the demystification of the patient's illness. By allowing the patient to remain in his own environment, the social costs to him are much reduced.

Disadvantages

The disadvantages of the use of medication for violent patients in an emergency situation include the numerous side-effects of the drugs themselves, that by and large, have already been mentioned. However, there are many more, for example sudden death, laryngospasm, respiratory distress, electroencephalogram changes, convulsions, tachycardia and arrhythmias, endocrine disturbances, agranulocytosis and so on. Although many of these are rare, they constitute possibilities to which nurses and doctors should remain alert.

Other disadvantages would include the difficulties of administering injections to violently struggling patients and the concomitant injuries that could be sustained. Although we have emphasised the necessity for physical control of a struggling patient prior to injection, sudden surges of movement can snap the needle leaving it embedded in the patient's muscle. In these cases, the attending physician may require a cut-down set to remove it when the patient is more settled. Damage to injection sites can also occur, as can excessive bleeding if veins or arteries are punctured.

These advantages and disadvantages are specific to the application of medications in the psychiatric emergency and do not cover the ethical considerations of this mode of restraint generally, which we have mentioned earlier in the chapter.

SUPPORTIVE ASPECTS TO EMERGENCY MEDICATION

As with all forms of human interactions, especially with psychiatric patients in crisis, the skills of mental health workers are drawn upon to ensure that the quality of the therapeutic engagement is maximised. When restraints are being applied, in all their variations from limit setting to chemical control, it is important to maintain an interactive style that fosters the therapeutic potential. Whilst using a body-belt on someone who is violent or forcing an emergency injection on someone, both forms of restraint are applied against the person's will, and in the first instance, patients often resent these approaches bitterly. However, the damaging impact of these forms of restraint can be minimised by a firm but compassionate approach.

There are three general areas of good practice; these include, firstly, promoting safety, secondly, effective communication and, thirdly, attention to daily needs.

Safety

The safety of the patient, fellow residents, visitors and staff is of paramount importance and everyone will appreciate a mature professional approach to ensuring it. Bravado is not necessary and can be extremely dangerous. Ensure that an adequate assessment takes place of the balance between safety and resources. The least restrictive method that is the most effective will ensure a satisfactory outcome for all. Staff running around, looking uneasy and furtively glancing in all directions do not portray a confident image. Therefore, promote calmness and ensure each knows his role and the appropriate signals for action.

Communication

Effective communication will ensure that all those involved are reassured. The patient should be informed of the events as they occur and needs to know that they are not punitive actions, but considered to be in the patient's best interests. As he regains internal control, this message should be reinforced and if he is cognitively intact, he should be informed as to required behaviours as he gains further control. Orientating the patient to time, place, self and events that have occurred should be undertaken sensitively with constant reassurance; the assessment of his response to this orientation is a good indicator of his mental state.

Attention to daily needs

Daily needs require attention. Acutely disturbed individuals may well have gone some considerable time without food or drink and may require both. However, these should be given under medical prescription if the patient is heavily sedated, as patients have asphyxiated on regurgitated food. Other aspects of daily living include attention to personal hygiene and toileting needs as, again, sedated patients can experience incontinence and this can be both demeaning and distressing.

All in all, these supportive aspects merely involve good nursing care which should be applied in these, often, difficult procedures.

FUTURE DEVELOPMENTS

Before we conclude this chapter, and Section Two of the book, we feel that it is necessary to mention some developments in the use of chemical control of the violent and aggressive individual.

Clozapine

The first concerns clozapine, which is briefly mentioned above, but which we would like to expand on here. Clozapine is an atypical antipsychotic agent that has become popular in treatment-resistant schizophrenia as it has relatively few extrapyramidal side-effects. Its antiaggressive action is receiving research attention with good early signs of success (Ratey et al 1993). Unfortunately, the drug has a high incidence of agranulocytosis so there is a need for very strict monitoring of the patient according to the pharmaceutical company's instructions. Although not all treatment-resistant patients benefit, there are good indications that many more than previously improve with the use of clozapine.

Mace

The second development concerns the use of chemical mace as a method for controlling violently disturbed mentally ill offenders (Conacher 1995). Chemical mace was developed in 1965 by the General Ordnance Equipment Company of Pittsburgh, Pennsylvania, USA. It is said that its 'active ingredient is alpha-chloroacetophenone (tear gas) dissolved in an organic, carrier-solvent compound at a concentration of about 0.9 per cent' (Weinberg et al 1970). This compound is compressed in a canister and is delivered in droplets similar to those in a commercial aerosol. It is sprayed into the face of the attacker. The effect of mace is the reflex closure of the eyes and the holding of breath to prevent inhalation; it causes instant immobility. No long-term injuries have been reported, to our knowledge, in the use of mace, but its use on psychiatric patients is fraught with ethical dilemmas. It has been used in prison psychiatric facilities in the USA, in which the extremes of violence and aggression have been reported. In the first instance it is used to incapacitate the violent person who is then given neuroleptic medication.

The impact of drug companies on psychiatry is profoundly influential and we would expect their research and development strategies undoubtedly to include the management of violence and aggression in the acute stages of crisis intervention. We can only anticipate that drugs will be developed to control disturbed persons in those moments of crisis when they become actively combatant.

CONCLUSIONS

We have seen throughout this chapter that the use of chemicals for the control and management of violent individuals can take a number of forms. We began by briefly outlining the use of drugs in the long-term therapeutic management of aggressive patients and then focused upon the early intervention of the psychiatric crisis by the use of PRN medication. However, it is the use of chemicals in the emergency situation that is the central theme of the chapter and this calls for accurate assessments of both the patient and the context in which the crisis is occurring. Planning and preparation for the emergency administration of drugs have been discussed and the central aspects of administration outlined. These included rapid sedation, rapid neuroleptisation, their side-effects and the documentation. Having set out some of the major advantages and disadvantages, we then discussed the role of mental health workers in developing therapeutic skills when administering emergency medications. Finally, we mentioned the development of chemical agents in the control of violent psychiatric patients.

In examining the moral principles involved in controlling and restraining violently disturbed persons, we have to resolve, at least to some degree, the difficulties of intellectual ping-pong with the pragmatics of application. Nowhere is this more the case than in the varying types of restraint highlighted in Section 2 of this book. Personal choices as well as hospital philosophies play a part in the thorny ethical dilemmas. Whether one prefers seclusion, physical holding, mechanical restraints or chemical control is a personal choice, however, as expressed by Conacher (1995): 'to a clinician who has been made at times deeply unhappy by some of the views expressed about psychiatry's role in a coercive system, this perspective, while it does little to resolve the many difficulties, seems one that is most in accord with the clinician's own inarticulate attempts to achieve some sort of resolution. In the end, it is one's own conscience with which one is forced to live' (p. 64).

SECTION 3

Corollaries of violence and aggression

SECTION CONTENTS

12

Serious situations

KEY POINTS

1. Serious situations can begin with very minor intentions.
2. The skills of negotiation lie at the heart of resolving these situations.
3. The hostage situation, the barricade and the protest can manifest as serious events but equally may be involved in minor situations.
4. The management of serious incidents has important lessons for the management of minor ones.
5. Certain situations appear paradoxical in relation to the patient population.
6. Learning about serious situations can aid our understanding of the dynamic of violence and aggression.

INTRODUCTION

In Section 2 of this book, we identified three phases of aggression in which various interventions could be applied. Although a good deal of overlap exists here, as the diversionary approaches in phase 1 can be continued during phase 2 and in some cases during phase 3, they have been grouped according to their major impact in each phase. During phase 1, there is a state of relative normality in which the potential for violence and aggression is always present but the general situation remains stable. During this phase, close observations are needed for an early appreciation of a deteriorating situation and the perception that something is wrong. Phase 2 is the phase of preaggression in which there is an awareness that a violent or aggressive encounter is more likely to occur and therefore interventions take on a more active format. We have pointed out that in many instances, in fact in more cases than not, violence and aggression are diverted during these interventions, although we tend not to be aware of many of these, as they usually go unreported. However, in some circumstances, violence does occur and an attack ensues. In these cases there are, generally, four main approaches to intervention: (a) isolation techniques, (b) physical restraints, (c) mechanical control and (d) chemical control, but it should be pointed out that there are many variations within each of these. We have also noted that these differing approaches are dependent upon the function of the host organisation, the imperative of the professional objectives and the type of person that is involved in the violent encounter. Furthermore, the situations are made even more complex by the social context in which they occur.

This final section comprises three chapters that deal with various corollaries of managing violence and aggression. The first chapter outlines various situations that can occur with violent individuals. The second discusses the types of injuries that can be sustained, the effect on staff in the form of job stress and the resultant condition of burn-out. The final chapter is concerned with how we learn from the experience of managing violence and aggression, which is of major importance if we are to progress to ever more successful interventions and the production of preventative strategies. The main message running through these three chapters is the importance of accepting the negative feelings that can emerge in managing violence, especially when things have gone wrong, and of using these emotions to gain positive insights. When we become aware of these negative feelings in others, it is crucial that we do not denigrate or condemn the person concerned, but instead offer support and positive regard for expressing such feelings.

In this chapter, we will first set out the major principles of negotiation, as this forms the basis of dealing with many of the situations that we then go on to discuss. Negotiation, like many other aspects of managing violence and aggression, is a skill that can be honed and refined but to some extent relies on the personality of the individual involved. Although many of the situations that we will briefly discuss are unlikely to be experienced by many staff in health care settings, *some* staff will most certainly meet them in the course of their careers. Furthermore, the principles of managing these situations, which are major events, are the same as those met in lesser encounters and therefore are equally important.

NEGOTIATION

Negotiation usually means that two, or more, parties confer with each other with a view to finding a compromise and agreement leading to a mutually successful outcome. For negotiation to take place, this requires both parties to have something that the other party desires, so that both have something to give as well as take. A further prerequisite for negotiation is that there must be some element of choice or decision-making capacity, otherwise what is taking place is not negotiation but more akin to a directive or an order. Thus, the dynamic of negotiation is fraught with tensions and conflicts based on a very fine, and delicate, balance of power.

The mechanism of negotiation refers to the actual bargaining of interests in which offers are made, their impact on the recipient is synthesised, and decisions are conducted in relation to the overall objectives. The negotiation process must then facilitate understanding between those involved and achieve an element of cooperation, whether they be individuals or organisations. Without understanding what each aspect of the negotiation means, not only to one's own party but also that of the other, there is a reduced likelihood of a successful outcome for all concerned (Kraus & Wilkenfeld 1993).

Types of negotiation strategy and behaviour

There are a number of negotiation and bargaining models that can be employed in real-life situations. Snyder & Diesling (1977) set out three types of negotiation strategies in a crisis situation. First was the *accommodative* approach; in this, there is a convergence of the party's negotiations towards a resolution via a sequence of proposals that involve demands, propositions and concessions. This approach is firmly rooted in the give and take perspective and relies on developing understanding of what is important for the other party. Second, there is the *coercive* approach; this involves an expression of firmness and may include delivering threats and warnings, and generally exerting pressure to influence the other. In this perspective, either party may adopt this stance. Finally, there is the *persuasive* approach; in this, there is no threat delivered but instead an appeal to the other party in order to influence its decision.

Leng (1987), on the other hand, set out certain behaviours that formed the crisis dyad; these included *fight*, whereby both parties adopt coercive strategies that exacerbate the conflict and result in violence. Others are *resistance*, where one party pursues a coercive strategy whilst the other stands firm; *stand-off*, in which both groups adopt strategies of firmness with neither party willing to give concessions; *dialogue*, which involves the accommodative approach above; and *prudence*, in which one party asserts themselves over the other leading to a quick submission.

Crisis bargaining

Another approach to negotiation, which has been particularly used in international conflicts, is crisis bargaining (Donohue, Ramesh & Borchgrevink 1991). This research contributes, along with others, to: 'develop communication strategies to deal with hostage takers who are mentally ill, those caught in the act of criminal activity, political terrorists, or prisoners involved in revolts' (Donohue, Ramesh & Borchgrevink 1991; p. 258). This model deals with how to turn a confrontative situation into a normative bargaining situation in order to facilitate arriving at a deal.

To develop this model, the above authors set out two key relational issues that maintain either a coercive or a cooperative relationship within the crisis situation: control and distance. Control is concerned with the negotiation of relational rights and obligations, and differs depending upon whether the situation is cooperative or coercive. In cooperative negotiation, the individuals involved subordinate some of their rights whilst sticking firmly to their role obligations, whereas in coercive situations, the individuals may reject the obligations of their role and augment their rights to achieve their objectives.

The second key relational issue is distance, which addresses the question of immediacy in both the physical and psychological use of space. The parties involved may, or may not, wish to remain in close physical proximity to one another. If the situation is cooperative, the parties may wish to remain in close proximity and give positive non-verbal cues. However, in conflict situations, the physical distance maintained may be greater and close proximity be quite stress provoking. Psychological distance is more concerned with the extent to which those involved trust each other, remain open and are honest. However, the physical and psychological distances are closely related in that the one usually accompanies the other.

Negotiated order theory

Developing out of this research, the negotiated order theory, which is rooted in symbolic interactionism, attempts to understand how the interactions within the negotiation framework sustain the social order (Donohue & Roberto 1993). The negotiated order theory is grounded on five basic principles. The first is that there are a set of limits that define the contextual properties of the interactions within the negotiation. Secondly, the setting of these limits is implicit and usually not attended to specifically, for example, one party may use humour to redefine these limits. Thirdly, the limits during negotiations are constantly being stretched and tested informally. Fourthly, the parties involved in the negotiations avoid issues that will threaten the accepted implicit limits. Finally, some limits are not negotiated. Although the model may well appear both complex and conceptual, the practical ramifications of this approach are an important contribution towards forming resolutions through negotiations. The framework establishes whether the parties involved are either moving against, moving away from, moving towards or moving with each other. Thus, it is a relational model.

Application of psychotherapeutic principles

The final model of negotiation that we would like to mention uses psychotherapeutic and self-psychology principles to analyse the negotiations (Feldmann & Johnson 1995). In this model, negotiation has similar properties to psychotherapy, in that it has developmental stages. The first stage is of the problems, *identification and exploration,* in which there is an emphasis on gathering essential information relating to the positions of the parties involved in the negotiations. Secondly, there follows *development of a working alliance*; although different from a therapeutic relationship, none the less, this requires those involved to establish an agreement to work together for the purposes of the negotiation. Thirdly, a *working through of goals* must occur; this involves each party understanding the other's objectives and the difficulties of meeting them, but successfully doing so. Finally, there is *termination,* in which surrenders are established either in the give and take of negotiation or as in the break in therapy.

In using self-psychology as an analytic framework for the negotiation of crisis situations, we are dealing with issues of empathy and transference reaction between the parties involved. These comprise elements of fragmentation and disintegration of the fragile self when exposed to stress (Feldmann & Johnson 1995). Thus, in negotiations it is important to focus on the types of self-object transferences that may be problematic.

In these negotiation models, we note a conceptual framework that can be used to inform the practical application of interpersonal behaviours during crisis negotiation. Or, put another way, the theory and practice conjoin to arrive at a resolution. They can be applied in many types of crisis and we now outline some situations in which negotiation can be employed.

SOME SERIOUS SITUATIONS

It is unlikely that many health care workers will face some of the situations that we mention here. However, for those that do, it is a devastatingly frightening situation that can often leave traumatic residue. Serious situations include hostage taking, barricades and protests.

The hostage situation

In our experience in high-security psychiatric hospitals, which totals over 40 years of practice, we have witnessed only four hostage situations. In one, the hostage was murdered, in another he was raped before being released, and in the other two the hostages were released physically unharmed. The important factor in hostage situations is, of course, the safe release of hostages; although there is an academically interesting argument about cost: benefit ratios, the rewarding of negative behaviours, etc., for those involved it is the practical aspects that are foremost in people's minds. Once a hostage situation has arisen, everyone involved – the hostage, the captor and the negotiator – are, to one degree or another, hostages to the situation and the valuable first lesson is, usually, that everyone involved wants a resolution.

As we have said above, negotiation has similarities to the therapeutic relationship but it is also fundamentally very different; therefore we would agree with Feldmann & Johnson (1995) that: 'mental health professionals should *not* serve as negotiators' (p. 210, emphasis in the original). This function should be undertaken by trained personnel within the police system. It is, however, appropriate for mental health professionals to act as on-scene advisors.

Neuro-physiological and emotional aspects

There are several dimensions to the hostage situation that require some degree of elucidation before we go on to discuss policy. The first is the biobehavioural dimension in which the physiological effects of adrenaline may well exacerbate an already tense situation. It is highly likely that these effects are being experienced by the hostages, the captors and the staff responding to the alarm. The extremely unstable inner state that results from these physiological effects adversely affects the logical flow of the thought processes. Therefore, the objective in the initial phase, often referred to as the *setting-in* phase, is to apply any technique that calms the situation (in biobehavioural terms, this is any intervention that shifts the balance of the autonomic nervous system from a sympathetic to a parasympathetic response – see below) (Gilmartin & Gibson 1985). Suitable techniques may include reducing audio stimuli, avoiding overactivity, reducing the rate of speech by speaking slowly oneself, and avoiding volatile words. The negotiator (in the initial stages, this is likely to involve local staff rather than a trained negotiator) should at this time attempt to settle things down and control the situation.

The second dimension involves two types of phenomena of which the negotiator should be aware. First, there is a phenomenon called the 'Stockholm syndrome', in which the hostages and captors develop positive feelings towards each other. Second, there is the 'John Kennedy' phenomenon; in this, the experience is of such a magnitude that there is a rapid learning generated by the sympathetic branch.

The third dimension in the biobehavioural model involves the induction of the parasympathetic responses. Any response the negotiator can elicit that will bring about parasympathetic action will increase the chances of a peaceful resolution. Eating, drinking, sleeping and smoking will all aid this reaction. The negotiator should gather information on the captor's biological clock to establish periods of hunger, sleepiness, etc.

Negotiation guidelines

Some basic rules in negotiation for hostage situations are set out in Box 12.1.

Box 12.1 Initial basic rules in hostage negotiation (adapted from Maksymchuk 1982)

Do not trade lives
Do not give drugs
Do not give weapons
Do not confront the captors
Do not give rewards
Do not argue or tell lies
Do not allow the situation to go mobile

Hostage situations involve setting down basic rules to establish the win–win result, in which there is a negotiation of the conflict, and avoid other outcomes such as:

- lose–lose, in which both parties learn to live with the conflict
- lose–win, whereby the negotiator avoids the conflict
- win–lose, by overcoming the situation with the use of force.

Being involved in a hostage situation is a crisis, but it is useful to note that hostage takers find themselves in this situation in an attempt to resolve another conflict. Organisations should have policy guidelines for hostage situations and also provide some advice for staff who may become hostages. This should include some of the items in Box 12.2. Following release, there is a need for a critical incident debriefing session to alleviate stress and reduce the possibility of individuals suffering post-traumatic stress disorder.

The barricade

The barricade situation may, in many ways, be similar to the hostage incident but it has one fundamental difference: the barricade can exist without a captive. Barricades can occur singly, with one person constructing a blockade against others, or may involve many individuals working together to form a barrier to access. There are a number of permutations to take into consideration, each one having a different interpersonal dynamic.

Box 12.2 Hostage situation policy guidelines (adapted from Powell 1991; Turner 1984)

If you are the initial contact:

Summon assistance	Ensure that help is on the way by whatever means you can
Calm and control the situation	Speak slowly and allow the situation to settle down
Set up some communication with captors	This may be verbal to begin with
Set up contacts	These should be both near the incident and away from it
Evacuate and isolate	Move others not involved in the situation away from it
Set down basic rules	(a) Understand that you cannot accept orders from the hostages unless it is immediately life threatening (b) you have no power to give in to any demands (c) use your powers of observation
Build rapport	(a) Keep calm (b) express empathy (c) be nondescript (d) encourage captor to talk (e) avoid accepting deadlines (f) help captor save 'face' (g) await trained negotiator (h) make no promises
Hand over	Give as much information as possible to the trained negotiator and include number of persons involved, geography, times, descriptions and causes

If you are the hostage:

Remain calm	Easier said than done, but vitally important to settle the situation down
Do not give up hope	Others are working hard for your safety
Do not show emotions	Overexcitement and hysteria will raise tensions and worsen the situation
Do not speak unless spoken to	Particularly in the initial phase as this will make the captors angry
Do as you are told	Be compliant to establish a degree of trust
Do not argue or make suggestions	This will make the captors angry and resentful
Relax	Although difficult, keep relaxed but also keep the captor facing you if possible
Keep alert	As release may be imminent
Rescue	In case of rescue attempt expect noise, flashing lights, smoke, etc. Lie flat on the floor. Guide rescuers to other hostages.

1. Single barricade – in this, one person builds a barricade against others. This situation may, or may not, involve threatened suicide. There is a need for great caution in this scenario. The biggest threat is complacency as there is a tendency to considering the situation non-threatening where a solitary person is involved. Negotiations should be initiated as early as possible.
2. Two-person barricade – if two people have constructed a barricade then they are likely to have similar causes and will quickly form a bond of defiance against intruders. They will bolster each other when needed and they will be able to take turns to remain vigilant whilst the other rests. Negotiations in this situation should be aimed at a resolution that satisfies both parties as one person left alone will be vulnerable to suicide.
3. Multiperson barricade – this usually occurs in the context of a riot and is a situation where there is a great deal of excitement and destructive power. Once established, the group dynamic becomes a self-reinforcing prescription of loyalty, which is difficult to penetrate. No member wishes to show any weakness and there is an interpersonal structure of sanction applied to any member who is seen to break ranks. Negotiations in these situations are usually protracted and are aimed at a resolution that either involves the entire group or works by getting individuals to surrender.
4. Barricade with hostage – we can see a number of possibilities in this scenario, with one or more captors taking one or more hostages. These can be very dangerous situations with the group dynamic justifying serious action against the hostages. Negotiations should commence as soon as possible and the situation should be personalised by the use of names rather than labels such as staff, patients or prisoners (Paterson & Leadbetter 1995).

The building of a barricade has a symbolic meaning as well as a practical use for the person concerned, so unless individuals are getting hurt, it is wiser to allow the energy to be expelled on building the barricade rather than fighting. As in the hostage situation, it is best to allow the incident to settle in and maintain calm so far as is possible. Observe for the construction of weapons and take note of safety factors, such as fractured gas pipes or torn electrical wires. Above all, remain very observant, as what initially appears to be a single barricade may well become a much more serious hostage-type situation.

The protest

Clearly the term 'protest' can be all encompassing and its manifestation can be far ranging. However, in all protests, there is a common element that needs to be addressed if resolution is to be achieved. No matter what form the protest takes, it contains a message, which is usually grounded in frustration. Protest is, generally speaking, undertaken when other more legitimate channels of communication have been thwarted, and attempts to address the particular issue have failed. Again, this has usually taken some considerable time to come to a head, with the frustrations mounting insidiously.

Another factor contributing to the understanding of protest is the issue of power. Protest occurs when the imbalance of power is considerable and the protestors consider themselves to be powerless and challenging the powerful. The issue of the protest may appear far removed from the protest itself, and thus considered irrational by some, but will be very logical to the persons undertaking the protest. Protestors may believe that they are confronting a system, an organisation or an ideology, but the victims involved will usually have little to do with the larger issues, and thus become depersonalised as nameless hostages. Herein lies the major strategy for managing such protests.

As we have said above, protests can take many forms but here we would like to outline three of the more common types.

1. The 'dirty protest' – the spreading of faeces is called 'scatolia' and this may be undertaken by some as a form of protest. Although scatolic behaviour is seen in many clinical conditions, from children with learning difficulties to elderly dementia patients, it is most common in prisoners as a form of resistance. However, it has also been reported to be relatively commonly used by protesting patients in both high- and medium-secure settings (Mason 1996a). The main issues surrounding scatolia are the health and safety aspects of those living in such conditions as well as those who must work in them.

The first stage in its resolution is to note the underlying message within the protest itself, which can be achieved through negotiation. The second stage involves negotiating the terms and conditions of removing persons from the fouled area and the cleaning of both themselves and the smeared faeces. In some establishments, there are specialist hygiene teams that undertake this cleaning, whilst in others the task falls to nurses and domestics. In any event, specialist equipment is needed and protective garments are an absolute necessity.

2. Rooftop incident – when patients or prisoners take to the roof as a protest, it causes disruption to large parts of the organisation. This can be a dangerous situation, as it is usually accompanied by destruction of the roof and the throwing of slates, tiles and bricks down below, which can cause serious damage to others. Therefore, there should be a 'sterile' no-go area set up around the building where no one should enter and this area should be as far as the thrown missiles extend. Staff should be allocated to strategic points to keep those on the roof under observation, and negotiations begun as soon as possible. With one protestor on the roof, there is a good chance of early resolution but when several are involved, the situation will tend to

be more drawn out as the group dynamic perpetuates loyalty between members and creates the fear of breaking ranks. Rooftop incidents need to be resolved through negotiation, rather than by force, owing to the obvious safety implications.

3. 'Smashing up' – this is a term used to describe someone who is engaged in destroying property, either his own or that of others. It is usually done in a rage and once again by people who are frustrated at something or someone. Decisions need to be taken about whether an intervention is needed or whether it is better to allow the person concerned to expel his energy on property. The patient may well be creating weapons by his destruction of property, or creating safety hazards, for instance by fracturing live electrical wires. In these situations, keep the person under observation and attempt to talk calmly to him. Try to engage him in conversation and keep him talking if possible.

Attempted absconsion

We will now turn our attention to another type of situation that may call for some form of restraint procedure. This is the attempted absconsion. Health care staff are often in charge of escorting patients who may be compulsorily detained under the Mental Health Act. They may find themselves escorting patients to court, to a general hospital for some form of treatment or outpatient appointment, or on rehabilitation trips to the local community. During these escorts, a patient may well attempt to abscond and require restraining. Undertaking this in the community, with other members of the public looking on, can cause additional problems. The public may not know that the person is legally detained and misinterpret the restraint as a fight or attempted mugging. They may intervene on the patient's behalf with the possibility of a serious situation developing.

To manage these situations, there are preventative strategies, which should be organised prior to the escort. For example, staff members should carry a warrant when escorting compulsorily detained patients; this can be shown to members of the public or to attending police officers. They should also carry an ID card to which a photograph is attached. Transport in the form of a car or bus should be nearby and the patient transferred to it as quickly as possible. If the patient runs away, then staff members should follow if they do not have responsibilities for others, leaving one member at a focal point to communicate with the authorities and pass both descriptions of the absconder and any information about any likely offences. If one staff member pursues the absconder, then he should merely track the patient and not attempt an intervention alone. People who are chased can become desperate and may turn on their pursuers or other members of the public. The alarm should be raised immediately and the police informed.

SOME PARTICULAR TYPES OF PATIENT

In this section, we would like to outline some types of patient who may be the cause of violent situations.

Suicidal patients in acute settings

It may not be readily apparent that a person who wishes to take his own life may become violent towards others. However, when one considers the desperation that is needed to terminate one's own life, when that attempt is thwarted by staff, the patient can become extremely angry and direct the violence towards those would-be helpers. When making contact with a suicidal patient, staff should take a few moments to survey him and their immediate surroundings to observe for potential weapons. During this 10 second survey (Lynch & Fuller 1994), staff should memorise the presentation of the patient so that at a later period, they have some baseline measure. Observe the patient's hands as these pose the greatest threat either when using weapons or when attacking others. Also, monitor the patient's eyes as they often look at a weapon before reaching for it and using it. A person who has made a suicidal attempt may be semiconscious and reacting to any drugs that may have been taken, so approach him with caution. Alcohol is associated with suicidal attempts so the patient may well be disinhibited. Check him for weapons and then do the customary assessment of airway, breathing and circulation. As the patient awakens, assess him for signs of violence and if he becomes aggressive then use restraining methods, or withdraw if more appropriate.

The basis of negotiations with suicidal patients is the establishment of trust; however, before this can be achieved, staff must engage the patient in a series of choices. When approaching the suicidal patient, ask him permission to do so, and once in close proximity, ask if you can take his pulse rate. This serves a number of purposes. First, it can help you evaluate the person's heart rate, for instance whether it is racing or irregular, second, it gives an indication as to the skin moisture and temperature, but third it establishes a physical contact that is based in caring and you will communicate this. The additional benefit of this physical contact is that if the person turns violent, then you have the quick ability to control at least one extremity. If possible, always take the pulse on the patient's dominant arm, which is usually the one without the wristwatch.

Homicidal patients

Fortunately, homicides in health care settings are rare; however, when they do occur, they are extremely traumatising for all those involved. Homicides can occur because of the patient's clinical condition, for example, in delusional or paranoid states, but may also be a result of organisational factors such as overcrowding, staff management, and poor response to non-compliance with medication (Ferracuti, Palermo & Manfredi 1993). They can also occur because of pacts being formed and gang cultures established in high-security psychiatric services and prisons. Furthermore, there can often be a sexual/relationship jealousy involving more than two individuals.

The permutations can include one patient killing one victim, two or more patients killing one victim, one patient killing two or more victims, and two or more patients killing two or more victims. There are also instances of staff members murdering both patients and fellow staff. However, here we wish to restrict the discussion to the patient group as perpetrators. When a homicide occurs, there is an understandable severe reaction from the public as well as the police, with an inquiry a common corollary. From the police investigation, the inquiry, and the coroner's inquest, there are attempts to establish responsibility for the homicide and to lay blame where appropriate. Therefore, it is vital to set up effective systems and policies prior to the occurrence of homicide in order to aid prevention, safeguard health professionals and secure vital evidence when these events do occur.

When a patient has been killed, it goes without saying that there must be a perpetrator to such a crime; therefore, the main thrust of managing the situation in the acute stages, involves safeguarding the scene of crime. Do not allow others into the area and avoid contaminating any forensic evidence. There will be a police investigation and, at the least, an inquest so documentation should be protected and computer files safeguarded. However, one also needs to consider the fact that there is a homicidal patient, possibly in the vicinity, who may be a threat to others or himself. Other wards should be informed and be requested to be on the alert for disturbed patients. Observe your patient group very closely for any unusual behaviours or anyone acting differently from usual. Do not give information away unnecessarily as this may jeopardise later testimony. The patient community may be restless about the loss of a peer or the perpetrator may be feeling guilty and acting strangely. Also remember that whoever has committed the homicide may well commit another.

Chronically assaultive patients

As we have observed many times throughout this book, generally those that engage in violent and aggressive behaviour are a heterogeneous group, and the response to them also requires a wide and varied repertoire. Chronically assaultive patients, again, can be a diverse group that may well include long-term prisoners with nothing left to lose, violent personality-disordered patients considered too dangerous to be released, grossly psychotic individuals, the sexually deviant, or those with severe learning difficulties. A common theme to these patients is the fact that they have usually been the focus of intense treatment down the years with many failed interventions (Chandley & Mason 1995) and tend to be considered non-responsive to treatment (Mason & Chandley 1995). They are also viewed as responsible for many assaults and injuries, and management strategies for them have generally been developed through trial and error. Whilst some patients are chronically assaultive because they plan and execute their violence and aggression to the maximum effect without remorse over the injury and suffering that they cause (Moran & Mason 1996), others have little control over their actions and are dangerous because of their impulsivity (Mason 1996b).

With chronically assaultive patients, there is a tendency to establish as safe a regimen as is possible, which involves a safety margin within acceptable parameters, and once established, to maintain this position indefinitely. In these situations, it is easy to see how there would be a reluctance to attempt different interventions or apply new approaches to managing such patients. This reluctance is related to the fact that as the patient has had a long history of assaults, he is presently being managed as safely as possible; therefore any new intervention could be viewed as threatening the safety factor. This attitude has been most commonly noted in the development of long-term seclusions and restraints (Mason et al 1996), and itself becomes problematic; the intransigence of the situation is the focus of a therapeutic endeavour usually referred to as 'decompression'.

The three principles that underscore the management of chronically assaultive patients are safety, control and therapy (Mason & Chandley 1995). Firstly, safety refers to the conditions in which the patient is managed; any action undertaken must bear in mind the safety of those operating the intervention, other staff or patients and, of course, the patient himself. We have pointed out previously, and would reiterate here, that staff should not expect to be, nor be expected by others to be, injured at work. Being attacked by another human being is *not* part of the job. Secondly, control must be established; allowing patients to rampage and hurt others is neither in their, nor in anyone else's, best interests. Such out-of-control behaviour merely leads to further problems including the build-up of negative feelings by others. Thirdly, therapeutic approaches must be maintained to prevent the stagnation of practice mentioned above. In our view, failing to be therapeutically effective is not a crime but failure to attempt it, is.

WEAPONS

Weapons used by people in health care settings are of two types, which in the acute phase may not require a differentiated response, but in the longer term, may well have vastly disparate management approaches.

The first type are the opportunistic weapons that just happen to be in the vicinity at the time, are produced from the destruction of property, or are created for the purpose *at that point in time*. Examples of these may be the ashtray picked up to be thrown, the leg of a chair broken in a fight, or glass broken deliberately to cause harm. In these situations, the attacker is usually out of control and completely disinhibited, and is likely to do something that he later regrets.

The second type of weapons comprise's those that the aggressor manufactures or fashions (or purchases) for the purpose of using as a weapon. These may well be guns or knives that are bought, or blades and stabbing implements that are made, or may be garottes or clubbing instruments. In these situations, the weapons are usually accompanied by a degree of rumination, planning and phantasising over the attack, and the perpetrator may well appear calm and determined.

Depending upon the weapon and circumstances, these types may require different responses. For example, the anger and rage that is usually associated with the weapon of opportunity, may require a calming or defusing strategy, whilst a person employing a weapon constructed for the purpose of using it, may respond to a rationalising approach, or it may be better to make a pre-emptive physical intervention. However, in both circumstances it is important to avoid heroics and to remember that, if safe to do so, you can take evasive action by escaping from the situation.

The principles of managing attacks using weapons are, again, dependent upon the type of weapon. If the attacker is armed with a gun, then compliance is the most appropriate strategy and the situation becomes similar to the hostage circumstances outlined above. If the weapon is a knife or club, then distance is the safest option. Keep your distance by travelling backwards, by turning and running, or by moving from side to side. Keep your head moving and attempt to get something between yourself and the attacker. If possible, acquire a defensive weapon of your own (e.g. a chair or shield of some description) (Rice et al 1989).

CONCLUSIONS

This chapter has been concerned with some of the more serious situations that can develop in some health care settings. These have included the development of the hostage situation, the construction of barricades and protest behaviours. Although these situations are rare, they can take many different forms, and the principles of managing them are common to many aggressive encounters in which a form of protest is being made, and you feel yourself powerless to the situation.

We have also dealt here with patients who attempt to abscond and require restraining in public, suicidal patients who become aggressive and those who commit a homicide. Again, these are fortunately rare, but when they do occur, they are paradoxes that confuse staff and can lead to decisions that later become the focus of criticism. It is the fact that their logic is inverted, that leads to such confusion. For example, the situations of the absconding patient who may receive assistance from the public, the suicidal patient who may turn his aggression outward to the person who prevents the suicide, and the patient who kills, may all contain unexpected twists that can lead staff to act unwisely or, more accurately, when judged to be so in retrospect. Finally, we have discussed both those patients who, for whatever reason, become chronically assaultive and require systems of management that are difficult to overturn, and those patients who use weapons to attack others. This chapter has been underscored by the principle of negotiation, which forms the basis of resolving many of these difficult situations.

Working in environments that can produce such serious situations as well as the more minor encounters is particularly stressful. Part of the problem is that a minor verbal altercation can become a physical assault, which can lead into an attack with a weapon and a serious hostage situation. We have no way, at the outset, of knowing which minor situation will lead to a major one, and this is severely stress provoking. In the next chapter we will deal with the corollaries of this.

13

Injuries, job stress and burn-out

KEY POINTS

1. Despite knowledge, skill and experience, injuries do occur.
2. Some injuries are accidental whilst others are deliberate.
3. Working in environments where violence and aggression occur is stressful.
4. Stress affects different people in different ways.
5. Burn-out can be caused by stress.
6. There are ways of managing burn-out to the benefit of all concerned.

INTRODUCTION

The nature of the world is such that it is safe to consider it a dangerous place. When human beings begin to interact with each other, as they invariably must, there is always a potential for conflict, tension and dispute. Our society is an ever-increasingly stressful one in which the strains of modern life combine to produce competing objectives, frustrations and both winners and losers. Decreasing space through increasing populations, and increasing demands in decreasing time, produce contradictions, impatience and disappointment. For some people, this can lead to withdrawal, burn-out and mental illness, whilst for others, it results in disinhibited behaviour, violence and aggression, and in extreme cases homicide. One can only imagine the depths of despair in the minds of Ryan in Hungerford, and Hamilton in Dunblane, as they walked amidst the vulnerable of our society and wreaked havoc.

Health services exist to aid those who suffer, in whatever way, and who, by dint of their ailment, must interact with those people providing such services. It is often ironic that those whom we are attempting to help, actually become the ones to assault us. From the angry person kept waiting in the outpatient department to the psychotic at the emergency psychiatric clinic, and from the bloodied drunken youth in the accident and emergency department to the drug-crazed prisoner in the prison hospital wing, violence and aggression emanates from those we wish to assist. We do not dismiss our own personal roles in contributing to their violence, nor do we excuse the operational strategy of the organisation as an augmenting factor in the production of aggression, but the fact remains that we are assaulted by patients that we are attempting to care for. Furthermore, we can actually become the target of assault not only directly from patients, but also from their friends and relatives, and the friends and relatives of any victims of a patient's actions. This leads us to another dynamic within the complex interplay of factors that construct the violence and aggression in all health care settings: our response to such assault.

It may seem an obvious statement to make - that when we are assaulted, it hurts. However, the pain of the reaction to the same injury differs, depending upon the context in which it takes place. It is true that the pain of the bruised flesh is the same no matter what its causation; what makes it different in different cases is the emotional distress that accompanies the injury. The component of this emotional response will probably include such personal attributes as: (a) the extent of humiliation felt, (b) the personal insult incurred, (c) the loss of 'face', (d) the trust that is broken, (e) the injustice that is perceived and (f) the desire for retribution. These aspects will be contingent on the perceived motivations of the attacker and the perceived responsibility that they have for their actions. For example, the mentally impaired child who impulsively issues the bruise is viewed differently from the 'psychopath' who plans the assault; similarly, the drunken youth who attacks you may be viewed to be qualitatively different from the psychotic who believes that you are the devil. It should be emphasised that in all these examples, the motivation for the assault may well be calculated and callous; however, our response to them is determined by how we *believe* they are motivated.

This chapter will deal with the issue of injuries that are sustained in health care settings as a result of assaults by patients and will include types of attack, the characteristics of both the attacker and the victim, the types of injuries that are sustained, and the cost in physical, emotional and financial terms. We will also discuss the issues relating to stress from both actual and threatened violence and the response of burn-out from working in such stressful environments.

INJURIES

Injuries sustained from assault have many contributing factors; it helps to break down these into subsections to further our understanding of this complex topic. These include contact time, staff experience, intent, and personal characteristics of both victims and perpetrators.

Assaults and professional groups

It is an obvious statement to make - that in order to be assaulted by a patient one needs to have contact with him. Therefore, the first issue to discuss concerns those professionals who have patient contact and the extent of time that this involves. Although there are other issues pertaining to the risk of being assaulted, for example, the personal interactive styles and the role of the professional as perceived by the attacker, these will be discussed later. Here, we wish to focus on patient contact time with professionals as the first factor.

There are few studies that report on attacks by patients in relation to professional groups; however, the few that do, tend to report high rates of assault. In a survey of 115 psychiatrists in the USA, 41.7% reported being assaulted in their professional lifetime (Madden, Lion & Penna 1976). A similar figure of 42% was reported in a study of psychotherapists in San Diego (Bernstein 1981), whilst response to a questionnaire identified a lower number of assaulted psychiatrists in Philadelphia, at 20.2%, which was similar to the 24.4% of assaulted psychiatrists in a London study (Hatti & Dubin 1982). These reports were from research on general psychiatric inpatient populations; however, we can see that once the patient becomes an outpatient, the risk of assault reduces dramatically, but again not solely because of the reduced contact time. Reid & Kang (1986) reported only 3.2% of 156 psychiatrists as being assaulted by outpatients. In a large forensic hospital in California, Carmel & Hunter (1991) reported 13% of psychiatrists as having been assaulted, whereas Larkin, Murtagh & Jones (1988), in an equivalent setting in Britain, found that out of 1144 incidents of violence over a 6 month period, there were no psychiatrists attacked, but that the majority of assaults were aimed at nursing staff.

In relation to other professional groups there is a general agreement that nursing staff are assaulted with a frequency equal to that of psychiatrists (Carmel & Hunter 1991; Haffke & Reid 1983) but that the other two main professional groups, social workers and psychologists, are assaulted less, even when taking into consideration that their contact time with patients is likely to be less than in the first two groups (Haffke et al 1983). Caution is needed in comparing these studies, however, as definitions of assault tend to differ, as does the equation used to measure contact time. Furthermore, other factors also have an effect on the risk of assault.

Assault and experience

There is some evidence that the risk of assault reduces as experience is gained, both for psychiatrists and nurses (Carmel et al 1991; Haffke & Reid 1983). However, why this is so is not clear. It may be that with experience more knowledge is gained, which results in more effective management of aggression, or that de-escalation becomes more effective, or that avoidance of violent situations becomes a skilled practice. In any event, experience brings an increasing stock of knowledge pertaining to violence and aggression whereby each new situation can be evaluated by its similarity to previous ones in which outcomes are known (see Typification in Chapter 14, p. 242). This brings confidence in managing the current situation being faced, and it may be that this is the factor reducing the risk of injury and assault.

Assault and intent

For those facing violent and aggressive individuals, there are three types of intent to cause injuries that should be considered. The first refers to injuries sustained when attempting to control the combatant, which are often quasiaccidental. That is, they may be injuries received from a person who is kicking and flailing his arms where the blow is not specifically directed or aimed at anyone. They also include injuries such as sprains and pulled muscles resulting from sudden exertion.

The second type of intent can be described as attacker's motivation to do harm to anyone involved in the current aggressive situation; this can also be viewed as multidirectional intent. In this scenario, the attacker wishes to do harm to anyone in his vicinity; it usually involves a loss of temper and extremes of anger and outrage. These situations are explosive and serious injury can be sustained.

Finally, there is the planned unidirectional intent mode in which the victim is chosen specifically, for whatever reason, and the assault is geared towards harm to that individual. This usually involves planning by the attacker, who may engineer a situation and have some control over the occurrence of the events. Some considerable time may be invested by the assailant in fashioning a weapon specifically for the purpose of causing harm to one individual. There is a festering, simmering, hatred being built up, and therefore, assaults resulting from this type of intent, are often lethal.

The importance of understanding the intent of assaults is that they may well govern our response to attempting to intervene and our reactions to being injured. For example, in the quasiaccidental intent, there is little we can do other than maintain a state of physical fitness and general good health. In the multidirectional intent, skilled procedures such as C&R techniques need to be brought into play. However, in the last, unidirectional, mode, it is the skills of psychiatric interventions that are at the forefront of preventative approaches. It is worth noting that the risks of injuries associated with responding to violence and aggression are greater when restraining procedures involve only physical force – there are less injuries when mechanical restraints are used (Hill & Spreat 1987). These authors also note that planned interventions were safer than was responding to an emergency situation.

Characteristics of victims and perpetrators

Victims

As in the section on 'assaults on professions', there are few studies that specifically refer to individual characteristics of victims. Most studies attempt to uncover such aspects as experience, length of qualifications, age, gender, ethnicity, etc. and usually have a comparison group of non-assaulted personnel. These studies then go on to report that males are more likely to be assaulted than females or that inexperienced staff are injured more than experienced ones (Carmel & Hunter 1991). However, what is missing from these types of studies are issues relating to the personal attributes and interactive characteristics of those staff who are assaulted. Assault is more likely, in our view, to be related to the extent of arrogance, brusqueness, aloofness, etc. of professional staff, coupled to issues of domination, power and coercion, rather than to factors such as age alone (Ruben, Wolkon & Yamamoto 1980).

Assaulters

The characteristics of those persons who assault others are, again, diverse and without a clear pattern, despite the fact that it is commonly reported that the person most likely to cause injury to another is a young, psychotic male. However, there are a number of features in which the increased rate of violence is noted. For example, in the presence of delusions and hallucination or in those persons with drug or alcohol intoxication.

The setting

We are all well aware that certain areas, or settings in life, are prone to be more violent than others and if we increase our vulnerability by putting ourselves in those areas, then we may expect or anticipate problems.

However, the issue is not always quite as simple as this in relation to health care settings. For instance, one would expect that those establishments who, by their nature, cater for patients exhibiting excessive forms of violence and aggression, would be extremely dangerous places to work. However, the reverse is often the case, as those establishments tend to operate systems that contain such outbursts of violence, have extensive experience in doing so, and educate and train staff in the various skills and techniques needed for these situations. Injuries are actually more likely to be sustained in acute general settings than in specialist forensic units (Hunter & Carmel 1992).

Types of injuries sustained

Definitions of injuries are difficult to delineate as the subjective experience of receiving injuries differs among individuals and cultures. However, one main categorisation used is to distinguish between: (a) mild physical harm not requiring medical treatment, (b) moderate physical harm requiring medical treatment, and (c) serious physical harm with considerable time off work or medical retirement. This, of course, is not entirely satisfactory as there are clear problems of interpretation across all three types. Another way of classifying injuries is by the extent of time taken off work, but again this can be misleading.

The types of injuries sustained in health care settings very much reflect whether the weapons used are opportunistic or are fashioned (see Chapters 8, 9 and 12); that is, injuries differ as a result of the type of weapon available. Therefore, another factor connected to weapon use will be the setting in which the assault takes place. For example, in a profile of trauma due to violence in a statewide prison population in the USA, Bragg et al (1992) reported that 1600 inmates were hospitalised over a 3 year period, and 19 different weapons were used from an array of cafeteria, workshop and office equipment. More than 50% of the injuries were sustained from being hit by a fist or kicked. The highest type of injuries were orthopaedic (31%), followed by nasal deformity and penetrating wound (both 18%). In a state hospital, Hanson & Balk (1992) claimed that the injuries ranged from scratches, bruises and abrasions to severe back and eye injuries. In Britain, Cembrowicz & Shepard (1992) reported on trauma sustained in an accident and emergency department in which the majority of injuries were as a result of being punched, kicked, grabbed, stabbed, scratched, slapped, headbutted, strangled and hair pulled, in decreasing frequency, and by the use of furniture and fittings, knives, wheelchairs, broken bottles, broken glass, scaffold poles, planks, scissors, stretcher poles, syringes and needles. Clearly, the types of injuries are extremely diverse, as are the types of weapon used.

Cost of injuries sustained

When counting the cost of injuries sustained in health care settings, again, we have difficulties in measuring differences in emotional, psychological, physical and financial terms. However, we can note the following:

- Emotional responses to injuries are particularly distressing and can last for long periods of time far in excess of any physical damage. There can be feelings of shame, fear and disbelief, which can have a traumatising effect on the social functioning of the victim.
- Psychological responses to injuries are also damaging as the victim's physical integrity has been threatened. Intense anger and helplessness can lead to worry and frustration.
- Physical costs of injuries include the pain, discomfort and often gross inconvenience that accompanies injury. There may well be permanent disfigurement with its psychosocial corollaries or there may be permanent damage, which handicaps the person indefinitely.
- In financial terms, violence is a costly business. There are few studies that have actually reported financial figures but the majority of published work in this area concludes that it is, indeed, costly. Of those that present actual figures, we see a wide range of costs. Lanza & Milner (1989) reported a total cost to their hospital over a 1 year period of $38 000, which by all accounts, is a relatively small financial burden. However, in a similar 1 year period, Hunter & Carmel (1992) reported their hospital's (forensic) loss as $766 290. Although the manner in which the loss is calculated differs, we can see the large amounts involved.

Practical issues

We do not wish to enter here into the first aid requirements in cases of injuries sustained, as this is adequately covered in numerous texts. However, there are some practical issues that should be mentioned in relation to injuries that are received. These include both underreporting and redress.

Underreporting

We have known for some considerable time that underreporting of assaults is a recurring problem in numerous health care settings (Lion, Snyder & Merrill 1981). There are a number of reasons for this, such as apathy, long-winded administrative procedures, difficult access to documentation, poor response from managers, minor injuries becoming the accepted norm, the possibility that it may be perceived as a performance failure, and the cultural expectations which sometimes belittle reporting of such injuries. We would emphasise in the strongest terms, however, that all assaults and injuries sustained whilst managing violence and aggression, must be recorded in the appropriate documentation and the correct records maintained. The reasons for this emphasis are that: (a) we need to highlight the existence and extent of the problem, (b) underreporting may lead to underresourcing, and (c) problems that may require compensation can occur at a later date, and without the adequate records, there is little chance of success.

Redress

The second practical issue concerns the pursuance of redress when one is assaulted or injured. If you are assaulted or injured in the course of conducting your professional duty, then a claim for compensation should be pursued through the appropriate channels, including the Criminal Injuries Compensation Board and Compensation Orders. Mitigation and extenuating circumstances are the business of the courts and tribunals, and are not the concern of the victim of assault. Although often difficult to pursue, because of the stringent conditions that must be met with mentally disordered persons who engage in violence, there is a need to maintain a degree of pressure to affect the law in these matters.

STRESS

There is a wealth of information, which is growing steadily, on stress in the health care workplace; for those who face violence and aggression as part of their job, this is an important area of concern. The first thing to note is the distinction between chronic stress and acute stress when managing violence. Acute stress occurs when there is a sudden crisis and a quick response is called for. Acute stress is short lived but very intense. On the other hand, chronic stress often lies hidden just beneath the surface of awareness. Working in an environment where there is a daily potential for violence and aggression, but without it actually occurring, produces an insidious state of anxiety that resides permanently within the person. This anxiety does not find a ready release and there is no satisfactory level of recuperation on days off. This is a most unhealthy working environment.

Models of stress

There exist various models by which we can understand the causation of stress, and inherently within these, are strategies for overcoming the negative effects of stress.

Exchange and communal orientation model

The first type of model is the exchange and communal orientation model, of which there are several variants; in this, a lack of reciprocity of social support from colleagues is considered to produce stress at work (Buunk et al 1993). In this type of stress modelling, the support relationships between peers and managers are considered to be a major influence on the production of stress-related negative symptoms (LaGaipa 1977). Walster, Walster & Berscheid (1978) suggested that in different types of helping relationships, the extent to which a person considers themselves to be undersupported, will dictate the level of perceived stress. In a similar vein, Greenberg & Westcott (1983) postulated a 'degree of indebtedness,' which was a negative affective consequence of being in a position to receive help, and argued that this contributed to the production of stress owing to the fear of being unable to repay such debt. What these approaches share in common, is the idea a social network in which workers can feel a relationship has become unequitable. In these stressful situations, the solutions therefore point to regaining some form of equilibrium within the social relations that have become tense.

Perceptual models

Another modelling cluster of stress theories comprises perceptual designs, which to one degree or another involve the evaluation of a situation that is perceived as threatening. The threat may, in fact, be either real or merely perceived; nevertheless, the perception of a threat causes stress. Lazarus & Folkman (1984) are the central proponents of this type of model; they believed that the appraisal of an imaginary threat could lead to more severe symptoms of stress than could that of a real threat, depending upon the perception of the observer. Feinstein & Dolan (1991) took this work further by investigating whether the extent of actual severity of the threat produced symptoms of stress in the longer term and showed that the initial reaction to the assault had the greatest influence on the end result. Poyner & Warne (1986) also developed a model of stress as a result of violence in the workplace setting. In their model, there was a focus on the type of violence that takes place rather than the outcome or consequences for the victim. However, conceptualising these dimensions to be distinguishable from each other is flawed in certain respects, as seen from a psychological viewpoint. Two other workers in this area have produced an exciting tranche of literature that has not only incisively critiqued extant models, but has also developed a practical model of staff appraisal of violent situations in the health care workplace (Whittington & Patterson 1995, Whittington, Shuttleworth & Hill 1996, Whittington & Wykes 1994a, b, unpublished work 1995, Wykes & Whittington 1994.)

Responses to stress

Responses to stress can be wide and varied – so diverse, in fact, that almost any sign or symptom can be attributed to a stressful reaction. However, they do fall into a number of distinct types.

Emotional, social and biophysiological reactions

An early classificatory system was that by Lanza (1983) who set out a basic category of reactions, which has been adapted below.

1. Emotional reactions, short term – these include such items as anger, fear, anxiety, helplessness, resignation, sadness, guilt, depression, shock, apathy, empathy, disbelief and dependency.
2. Emotional reactions, long term – these include anxiety, anger, fear of the patient and sympathy for the patient.
3. Social reactions, short term – these include changes in personal relationships with coworkers and problems in returning back to work.
4. Biophysiological reactions, short term – these include startle responses, disturbances to sleep patterns, soreness, aches and headaches.
5. Biophysiological reactions, long term – these include body tension and general soreness.

Denial and intrusion phases

Horowitz (1986) argued that there is a general response to stressful events that is manifested irrespective of the type of situation that is encountered. Grouping symptoms together as a syndrome, Horowitz (1986) claims that there are two phases to this response.

Phase one – denial – includes:

- perceptual symptoms – such as attention deficits, inability to assess stimuli appropriately, forgetfulness, daydreaming
- ideation-processing symptoms – e.g. rigidity of thought, fantasy construction and distortion of meanings
- emotional symptoms – e.g. flatness of responses, feelings of numbness and low mood
- somatic symptoms – e.g. signs of tenseness, anxiety and agitation
- extremes of reaction symptoms – e.g. those ranging from overactivity to total withdrawal.

Phase two – intrusion – includes:

- attentional symptoms – e.g. hypervigilance, increased startle reactions, disturbances of sleep and dreams
- consciousness symptoms – e.g. thought intrusion, obsessional behaviours, nightmares and repetitive thoughts
- ideation-processing symptoms – e.g. tendencies to overgeneralise, be preoccupied with specific issues, and to be confused and disorganised in other areas of life
- emotional symptoms – e.g. sudden surges of emotions
- somatic symptoms – e.g. sudden desires towards fight or flight responses.

The response cycle

Wykes & Whittington (1994) have produced a comprehensive grouping of responses, in terms of both their specific symptoms and their response cycle. These include:

- specific symptoms such as anxiety, fears and phobias, cognitive effects, guilt and self-blame, and anger and morbid hatred
- response cycle – the three phases of impact, recoil and reorganisation.

These authors' work is a comprehensive account of the reactions of staff to stressful situations in health care settings and is strongly recommended as further reading.

Stress debriefing

When stress occurs, it cannot be allowed to continue. Two basic approaches are required to combat its negative effects. The first approach is to identify the source of the stress and to remove it, alter it, or change its direction where possible, then to learn from it to ensure that future sources of stress are reduced or eliminated. The second approach is to ensure that those persons suffering from stress are aided in the process of recovery. In this section, we will briefly outline three methods of stress debriefing – psychological autopsy (PA), critical incident stress debriefing (CISD) and psychiatric stress debriefing (PSD) – but would also point out that there is some degree of overlap between them.

Psychological autopsy (PA)

This approach was initially developed in America in response to suicides. It is used to investigate the reasons why the person committed suicide, to establish whether certain indicators had been missed, or not acted upon by others, and to examine the extent to which interventions could have been more effective. The PA usually takes place in an informal setting without undue pressure on attenders to account for themselves. However, the PA is conducted in two phases: a cognitive phase and an affective phase, in which an in-depth picture of the life and death of the patient is constructed. Although the primary focus is on the suicide victim, the 'significant others' in the patient's life and death are involved in the process. This approach has a learning emphasis in order that lessons for future care can be developed, but there is a second, recuperative, focus in helping survivors overcome their grief (Cooper 1995; Schneidman 1969). Although developed for suicides, it has been used in other psychiatric crises (Beskow, Runeson & Asgard 1990).

Critical incident stress debriefing (CISD)

This approach to stress debriefing was initially developed in the military (Samter et al 1993) as a planned strategy to analyse the facts of an event, the thoughts of those involved and the feelings that are engendered about an incident. CISD is used to help military personnel come to terms with combat incidents through a detailed analysis of the facts and through supporting the people concerned to reintegrate into the lifeworld of the soldiers, thereby helping to reduce undesirable emotional activity. CISD was developed as a therapeutic endeavour and there is a heavy emphasis on recovery of those afflicted, using an exploration of facts and feelings and an educational aspect (Cooper 1995). CISD adopts a seven-staged approach that includes: (a) introduction, (b) fact finding, (c) thoughts, (d) reactions, (e) symptoms, (f) teaching and (g) re-entry.

Psychiatric stress debriefing (PSD)

This approach is based on a merging of the PA and the CISD methods (Cooper 1995). The PSD approach involves an analysis of the precrisis functioning, the reaction to the crisis or the level of disruption, and the resolution to the state of equilibrium. The setting for the PSD is much more structured than in the former two approaches and there are few restrictions on time (Clark & Friedman 1992). The facilitator may be a mental health professional or a skilled para professional, but in any event, they must be familiar with the setting in which the crisis is set. The debriefing protocol follows the same stages set out in CISD above and involves (Cooper 1995):

1. Introduction – this includes an announcement of the purpose of the group and the setting of ground rules including such aspects as confidentiality, honesty and the avoidance of criticism.
2. Fact-finding – this involves describing the event from each member's perspective, establishing prodromal signs, identifying the extent of provocations, providing an explanation of how it started, who was involved, how they reacted and how the situation was resolved.
3. Thought stage – this is voluntary but the quest is for initial thoughts and subjective interpretations. It encourages members to get in touch with their feelings and allows for exploration.
4. Reaction stage – in this stage, a discussion takes place regarding the reactions of members. This can be a highly charged experience and needs careful management.
5. Symptom stage – this involves an identification of signs and symptoms of stress and should be geared towards returning the person to the precrisis level of functioning.
6. Teaching stage – this involves a skilled facilitator employing a thera-

peutic relationship. Teaching members about grief reactions, transference and countertransference issues, and stress management is undertaken in this stage.

7. Re-entry stage – this involves finalising of any further questions and assessing the success of re-entry into normal routines.

These, then, are three approaches to practical stress management and are useful as learning aids. However, they should not be regarded as fixed entities, but should be dynamically employed in a number of situations and adapted where necessary.

BURN-OUT

The task of facing violent and aggressive persons, in both the acute phase of hands-on approaches to specific events and the chronic phase of long-term threat, is clearly a stressful one. Furthermore, when this task often leads to injuries, then the combined pressures can lead to the condition of burn-out.

Definitions

Burn-out is a term that emanates from the field of sport; it describes a situation in which the performance of athletes fades after a promising start. They become exhausted following strenuous exertion. It has now been adopted into the jargon of many walks of life such as teaching (Belcastro, Gold & Hays 1983) and industry (Nagy 1985), and is used as well, in a number of health care settings, for example, in physiotherapy (Taylor, Sinclair & Wals 1987) and cardiovascular medicine (Grayboys 1986). However, it is in the area of mental health that the majority of research is focused. A number of authors have attempted to define the concept but there is little agreement between them. Table 13.1 shows the current range of definitions. This list shows the extent to which the meaning of the term can be adapted by individual authors to fit the particular paradigm from which they view the world. The question is, to what extent can we find common themes throughout them?

Maslach (1982) suggested that there are three central traits to burn-out. Firstly, it appears to occur at an individual level; secondly, it is understood as an intrapsychic experience involving feelings, attitudes and motives; thirdly, it is viewed as a negative experience with negative consequences. However, these dimensions lacked substance, so Starrin, Larsson & Styrborn (1990) produced an alternative 'Common list'. These authors claimed that another area of agreement was the notion of exhaustion, which was described as a loss of energy, weakness and tiredness and could be explained in physical terms or in psychological terms. A second area of agreement that these

Table 13.1 Definitions of burn-out (adapted from Starrin, Larsson & Styrborn 1990)

Study	Definition
Maslach & Jackson (1978)	The loss of concern for people with whom one is working (including) physical exhaustion (and) characterised by an emotional exhaustion in which the professional no longer has any positive feelings, sympathy, or respect for clients or patients (p. 3)
Freudenberger & Richelson (1980)	State of fatigue or frustration brought about by devotion to a cause, way of life, or relationship that failed to produce the expected reward (p. 13)
Cherniss (1980)	A process in which a previously committed professional disengages from his or her work in response to stress and strain experienced on the job (p. 18)
Edelwich & Brodsky (1980)	A progressive loss of idealism, energy and purpose experienced by people in the helping professions as a result of the conditions of their work (p. 14)
Pines & Aronson (1981)	The result of a constant or repeated emotional pressure associated with intense involvement with people over long periods of time (p. 15)
Veninga & Spradley (1981)	A debilitating psychological condition brought about by unrelieved work stress (p. 6)
Melchior et al (1996)	A syndrome of emotional exhaustion, depersonalisation and reduced personal accomplishment that occurs among individuals who do people work of some kind (p. 695)

workers found, was a negative shift in interpersonal interactions between people – for example depersonalisation, a lack of respect for patients and loss of idealism. Furthermore, they gave precision to Maslach's earlier third dimension mentioned above by claiming that this area of agreement entails: 'a negative attitude to clients, and the loss of idealism. Most discussions of this dimension emphasise its movement in a negative direction over time – a movement which is sometimes also characterised as a change, development or accumulation' (Starrin, Larsson & Styrborn 1990, p. 86).

Signs and symptoms

The signs and symptoms of burn-out overlap considerably with those of stress and can be equally wide and diverse. The reason why the response to burn-out can vary so much is that the response to stress can affect different people in different ways. This has caused some considerable controversy in the literature over whether such a syndrome as burn-out can actually be categorised as such. Box 13.1 identifies some of the major signs and symptoms of burn-out and it can be seen that the list is quite lengthy, but not exhaustive. This diversity of signs of burn-out is particularly problematic at an academic level; however, most staff working in the clinical area apparently know burn-out when they see it (Starrin, Larsson

Box 13.1 Some signs and symptoms of burn-out

Asthenia	Taking problems home	Loss of purpose
Headaches	Cynicism to patients	Dissatisfaction with job
Insomnia	Loss of temper	Physical exhaustion
Excessive self-confidence	Low efficiency	Increasing accidents
Boredom	Withdrawal from contact	Fatigue
Holding grudges	Increasing sick leave	Resistance to change
Depression	Hopelessness	Lack of dedication
Loss of interest	Loss of energy	Alcohol and drug abuse
Insensitivity to coworkers	Helplessness	Dislike of line-managers
Emotional exhaustion	Loss of idealism	Irritability

& Styrborn 1990). The common threads are, as mentioned above, a change in personality style from positive, motivated and enthusiastic to negative, demotivated and unenthusiastic.

In professional health care areas, where the acute management of violence and aggression is part of a daily potential occurrence, burn-out can not only jeopardise the person concerned, as the condition alters perception, slows reactions and reduces the capacity to deal with situations effectively (Braithwaite 1992), but can also affect those other staff who must take on the added work and responsibility of someone who is not performing up to standard. Furthermore, it is an added stress for the patients, who may become even more violent and aggressive as a result of an ineffective interaction with a victim of burn-out. What is clearly needed with a situation of burn-out is a strategy to alleviate the problem as a matter of urgency. However, before we look at alleviation, we need to address the issue of causation.

Causes

As with signs and symptoms, the list of causative factors of burn-out can also be wide and diverse (Box 13.2). However, again we can see common themes appearing in the list. For example, lack of support seems to be a major theme, whether this is peer group support or managerial support. A discrepancy between expectations and the ability to achieve fulfilment is another. Insufficient skills and knowledge to deal with aggressive patients is a third.

Dealing with burn-out

A solution will involve addressing the causative factors listed in Box 13.2. The first step, however, is the most crucial, and involves establishing an awareness that a problem actually exists. This is as much the case at an individual level as it is at an organisational one. If there is resistance to facing the problem, then the task is immeasurably more difficult. The following list gives some indicators of change that may need to be addressed.

Box 13.2 Some causative factors of burn-out

Increased patient caseloads	Lack of supervision	Scarce social support
Unfair promotion practices	Long days with few breaks	Patients who refuse treatment
Lack of positive rewards	High-stress environments	Lack of positive feedback
Insufficient staff	Restraining patients	Abuse from patients
Lack of interest from managers	Lack of career opportunities	Possibility of assault
Conflicts of role	Work overload	Overtime
Gap between aspirations and fulfilment	Status frustration	Deliberating whether actions will have support
Dealing with emotionally demanding patients	Lack of autonomy	Shiftwork

a. Individual changes that can be made include:

- make an effort to have interests outside of the job.
- take a holiday.
- attend workshops, seminars and conferences.
- arrange a personal action plan (strengths, weaknesses, opportunities, threats).
- organise supervision.
- set yourself realistic and achievable objectives.
- change your job if possible (internally or externally).

b. Organisational changes include:

- set realistic goals.
- set up support groups.
- give positive feedback.
- arrange for time-out.
- break routines.
- evaluate staff and arrange support training.
- provide job enrichment.
- plan careers.
- change authority structures if possible.
- engage staff members in decision making.
- allow self-management as far as possible.

CONCLUSIONS

We have seen in the early part of the book that the quest for knowledge and understanding of violence and aggression is a major concern for those working in settings in which the potential for harm can occur. As the book developed, we saw how the skills of all the varying management techniques were of great concern, especially in the acute phase when violence actually occurred and staff were involved in hands-on interventions. Now, as this book draws to a close, we have dealt with the major worries of injuries, stress and burn-out, which are, to one degree or another, results of 'things going wrong', as they invariably do. This statement is not intended to apportion blame, which it is sometimes appropriate to do, but to point out that the vagaries of human nature are such that all eventualities cannot be planned for, and we are left with the continuing quest to learn from each experience. This is the focus of the final chapter.

14

Learning from experience

KEY POINTS

1. The human mind has the ability to reflect upon itself.
2. There are a number of strategies to aid us to learn about violence.
3. Reviewing violent and aggressive incidents will help us understand them and contribute towards preventing other encounters.
4. Developing a learning culture is central to progressive practice.

INTRODUCTION

In the last chapter, we discussed the three central issues of injuries, stress and burn-out as the major problems for staff when managing violence and aggression. Although set out independently, these three areas are clearly interlinked and affect each other to one degree or another. Receiving injuries, however minor, can and does create stress leading to burn-out; similarly if someone suffers from burn-out then they are more susceptible to being injured. Therefore, strategies for avoiding these are a major concern for all those involved in managing violence and aggression, including those functioning in support roles, as well as those at the front line. We cannot expect merely to react to each new episode of violence and be eternally shocked and saddened by the injuries sustained. Rather, a proactive mode of thinking and action is needed to ensure that both theory and practice are developmental, and that environments are as safe as is humanly possible. That is, they should be safe in terms of physical layout, sufficient resources and clinical procedures. For this to occur, we need to learn from experience.

The Confucian adage 'a fool learns from his own mistakes: a wise man learns from the mistakes of others' will not suffice for our work in the management of violence and aggression. We will argue that learning takes many forms and is set within a discourse and a context that must be geared towards critical appraisal of practice, policy and procedure conducive to this learning. We will suggest that the personal learning from experience is a central tenet of development, and rather than 'a fool learning from his own mistakes', we will emphasise that true wisdom begins with this private reflection of personal experience. However, we will also agree that a 'wise man learns from the experience of others' as it is our contention that both types of experience should work together in a symbiotic manner, feeding each other and growing together. Taken apart, both are weakened, but united, they provide a profoundly influential mode of learning.

In this final chapter, we will set out the mechanics of learning in which reflexivity and typification will be outlined. This theoretical perspective will offer a basis for the establishment of a more practical endeavour such as engaging research, undertaking clinical supervision, formulating educational strategies and developing nurse–patient relationships. However, even with the best strategies, events do go wrong, and violence and aggression do occur, and in these situations, it is important that we review the situation accordingly. This will involve such approaches as postincident reviews, multidisciplinary working, and analysis of the contributing factors to violent encounters, the role of staff, and the lessons to be learnt following the event. A learning culture must be developed and can include both formal and informal approaches. Finally, we will highlight future directions in the management of violence and aggression before drawing overall conclusions.

MECHANICS OF LEARNING FROM EXPERIENCE

In simplistic terms, learning involves a series of steps that include observation, practice and evaluation. However, each step consists of very complex processes that must be undertaken for successful learning to be achieved. For appropriate observation to take place, there must be a series of judgements about what is going to be observed. These judgements emanate from one's previous experience and forms of knowledge. Action is operationalised repetitively in order that the process is smoothly enacted. This may entail subdividing the process into a series of successive operations (as in learning to drive a car), which are then rehearsed until the overall performance is achieved. This performance is then evaluated in relation to the objectives of the action, which involves reflecting upon the performance in relation to other performances. Such appraisal is undertaken by critical analysis, by the actor as well as the audience. Thus, we can begin to see a multifarious relationship formulating the notion of learning from experience.

Reflexivity

The first major theoretical problem we turn our philosophical attention to, is the notion of reflexivity. A great deal of our lives is based on routine, including our working lives. If this were not the case, our brain functioning would be so awash with contradictory deliberations concerning the most basic everyday procedures, that we would soon become 'frozen' in inaction. However, in developing our minds, and thus our behaviours, which in this instance concerns a set of actions involving learning from the violent outburst, there is a necessity to focus our attention on our specific thought pattern. This thought pattern involves the reflecting back of the experience of the individual upon himself in order that: 'the whole social process is thus brought into the experience of the individuals involved in it' (Mead 1934, p. 134). In this reflexiveness, the external social world, and its events, are brought into the experience, which then enables the person to appreciate the attitude of the other from this social world. By this process, the individual is in the position to adjust himself consciously towards the experience, and to revise the consequences of this reflexive process in any social situation in light of the adjustments made. This ability for reflexivity, then, not only enables the 'bending back' of the experience on the individual but also the 'bending back' of the experience of 'bending back' in relation to any adjustments made to the original bending-back experience (Mead 1934, p. 138).

In practice, this reflexivity entails making judgements about certain aspects of a personal experience of a violent encounter, and analyses in the form of questioning rather than making statements. Thus, the mode of reflexivity is an interpretive one in the form of an inner dialogue between possible questioners. There is no one single interpretation established from an external source but rather a series of possible interpretations from numerous internal conflicts, tensions and contradictions. The ability to engage in this reflexivity is governed by the person's aptitude for shelving taken-for-granted explanations and opening up one's mind to other, possibly uncomfortable, explanations. This, then, forms the basis for adapting one's behaviour in response to the experience of violence, or, as Winter (1989) put it: 'by showing that a statement is grounded in reflexive interpretive judgements, rather than in external facts, I make it possible to review other possible interpretive judgements concerning that statement, and thus to envisage modifying it' (p. 43).

The 'stock of knowledge'

The second aspect of theory we wish to address is typification, which is concerned with how we perceive violent situations and arrive at decisions on how to manage them. At any moment of time, we have available to us a growing 'stock of knowledge' pertaining to all life events, as when experiencing consciousness, every moment adds to our knowledge. The 'stock of knowledge' specifically relating to the management of violence and aggression also grows with every experience of these situations. For example, as we mentioned in earlier chapters of this book, we have all managed encounters in the school playground, sports fields, pubs and clubs, and every encounter has contributed to our 'stock of knowledge'. Thus, this bank of experience is constantly growing. Of course, every new moment is different from the previous one and no two moments are entirely the same. Similarly, every violent encounter is different from all others and no two aggressive incidents are actually identical.

Zones of relevance

To turn our attention to specific features of an experience requires those aspects to be relevant to us. These are known as 'zones of relevance'. There are said to be four main regions. Firstly, there is the zone of primary relevance, which can be immediately observed by us, and to some degree, controlled or dominated by us, by our actions upon it. Secondly, there are other fields not controlled by us, but which are important as they furnish information immediately connected to the primary zone. Thirdly, there are zones that, for the moment, are not relevant to us but which could become so, should changes occur. Finally, there are zones that are, and will remain, totally irrelevant to us as no changes will occur in them that influence our other zones. This last zone is the region of blind belief.

Typing of experience

As we said, all experience is unique; even an experience that recurs is not truly the same, simply because it recurs. It is the similarity to the previous experience that recurs, not the actual experience itself. However, when we experience an aggressive encounter, we can say that it is similar to a previous encounter because certain aspects of it are comparable, and by identifying the similar features, we can anticipate certain behaviours. Like objects, social situations can be put into 'types' in which one set of circumstances is deemed to be like a previously experienced set of circumstances. This then gives us the experience that one violent encounter is typical of another violent encounter, in which certain events occurred, and which could, typically, occur again. Thus, this system of relevancies and typification gives us the frame of reference for structuring the experience and formulating the response to it. However, it should be remembered that, as with the ever-changing moments, the 'stock of knowledge' also changes, as does our typification. Therefore, we can respond differently in similar situations in response to the changing events.

LEARNING STRATEGIES

There are, of course, many ways of learning about the management of violence and aggression. However, in focusing upon specific learning strategies from a practical point of view, we feel the following are worthy of note.

Research

Research is generally divided according to the natural and social scientific paradigms, or quantitative versus qualitative analyses, or 'hard' and 'soft' data approaches. Although we can benefit significantly from both these scientific paradigms, within which there are many different methods, we would here like to outline the case for action research.

Action research is based on the Kurt Lewin premise that: 'research that produces nothing but books will not suffice' (Lewin 1946, p. 36). It is a research approach that is grounded in the practice that is being studied and, as the name suggests, is about creating change or developing the potential for change. Action research has been defined as: 'a strategy for using scientific methods to solve practical problems in a way that contributes to general social science theory and knowledge' (Rapoport 1970, p. 499). The problem for action research is that it exists within the poles of the theory–practice divide, a traditionally amorphous, boundless and abstract region that is used for those occupying the extremities to keep the 'worlds' apart. The solution for action research is that it pulls both theory and practice into one conjoint processive activity. This embroils the enterprise in a state of affairs, or social inquiry, in which the theory and practice are inextricably entwined, affecting each other, often asymmetrically, and each complimenting the other in a dynamic progression.

The central tenet of action research is the cyclical nature of research constantly being folded into the practice under investigation. It is not only research *on* action, it is research *in* action. Action research has a cyclical structure in which the stages consist of analysis, fact finding, conceptualisation, planning, execution, further fact finding or evaluation, and then a repetition of the cycle. Describing the 'moments' of action research, Kemmis & McTaggart (1982) emphasise the four fundamental facets of the cycle: the *plan of action* designed to improve practice, the *act of implementation*, the *observation of the effects* of the action in the context, and the *reflection* on those effects forming the basis for further planning.

Supervision

Another concept that contributes significantly to the process of learning from experience is supervision, which includes a number of closely interrelated concepts including clinical supervision, mentorship and leadership. The underpinning theme for all these supervisory approaches is pedagogy, or the role of teaching.

Clinical supervision

Clinical supervision is a 'formal process whereby a student liaises with a more experienced practitioner in order to learn and refine therapeutic skills through the use of case material' (Rolfe 1990, p. 195). The supervisee meets on a regular basis with someone experienced in the field who supervises and evaluates the work undertaken. There are a number of models of clinical supervision, too numerous to enter into here; however, the underlying concept in them all is the relationship between the supervisor and the supervised in the learning process. This should be based on mutual trust, honesty and respect, which is underscored by confidentiality, with an exploration into the positive and negative aspects of clinical practice. It is a process that is not too dissimilar to the research method and is: 'qualitative in nature ... [and] ... can be compared with a research activity, an investigation about the interaction between people in a defined context' (Severinsson 1994, p. 274). It is hermeneutical in nature through its processes of interpretation of human interactions, and emancipatory in liberating restrictive impressions that are limiting evaluative operations. Done correctly, clinical supervision can offer a valuable approach to analysing violent and aggressive encounters in which feelings and values can be explored, interpreted and evaluated. This can provide a good learning exercise.

Mentorship

However, there are other supervisory models, as mentioned above, and two will be briefly mentioned here. The first refers to mentorship, which is defined as: 'a kind of learning through a planned teaming of two persons – one who is more knowledgeable, or more experienced, than the other' (Severinsson 1994, p. 274). Again, this is a pedagogical approach but it should be emphasised that this does not mean 'superior–subordinate positioning'. Mentorship is undertaken to provide role modelling and to encourage the exchange of information based on a relationship to establish self-esteem and job satisfaction.

Leadership

Finally, leadership should be mentioned in relation to the perspective of learning from experience. Although leadership can have both negative and positive responses from the same constructs (e.g. the creation of subordination, the execution of power and the capacity to convince others), it is the leader's behaviour, personal qualities and ability to form relationships that determine whether he will gain respect. The power of leadership qualities in learning about violence and aggression cannot be overemphasised and, given the formation of mutual respect, can constitute the basis of sound exploration.

Education

Education is a broad term that may encompass many types of learning from experience, including teaching, training and experiential approaches. However, we would like to make a basic distinction between formal and informal educative strategies. We cannot avoid the fact that for most of our conscious lives, we are gaining experiences and learning about our world, as outlined in the growing 'stock of knowledge' above. However, education becomes of central importance when we use it as a tool to focus upon a specific aspect of our world, (in this instance, the management of violence and aggression).

Formal education would include structured programmes for the management of violence and aggression held in recognised centres; in these, there would be a planned curriculum and a syllabus of study. There may also be evaluative processes to assess students' development. However, as important as these are, it is the informal strategies that we wish to focus upon here. Often, the luxury of joining recognised courses is not readily available and we need to address the fact that it is crucial that those staff so affected, adopt an educational spirit to inform themselves and others about managing violence and aggression. This can be achieved informally in the following ways:

1. Reading – there is an ever-growing volume of published material on violence and aggression and it cannot be overemphasised how important it is to keep up to date with this material. There should be regular visits to the library to keep abreast of recent publications and, most importantly, the most recent research. If photocopies are available, then these should be passed on to colleagues once you have finished with them. Most professional groups put some time of the working day or week aside for reading purposes and nurses should adopt this strategy as part of their professional development. Also, familiarise yourself with computer databases that allow you to search the literature and access as many previous publications as possible.

2. Writing – once you have familiarised yourself with the literature, you need to analyse it carefully and have a good command of the issues. It may be surprising to some, how educational it can be to attempt to set down on

paper, ideas about an issue, especially when part of the writing involves analysing many authors' works. Like reading, writing should be part of your daily/weekly work, and publishing material, part of your own professional development. Of course, it is a skill to be learnt and it may be helpful to form writing groups so staff members can assist each other.

3. Teaching – again, it may be surprising to some to discover how teaching others focuses the mind on a particular issue. Often, confusing material becomes clear when it is necessary to inform others about it. The teaching can deal with various aspects of violence and aggression and be aimed at students who are on placements, or towards colleagues, as part of their development programme.
4. Talking – debate is one of the most fruitful approaches to education and can be valuable in providing insights into many aspects of the management of violence and aggression. The forums could be small debating circles, workshop presentations, seminars and the more formal conference speeches.
5. Thinking – focused thinking on specific aspects of violence and aggression can help unravel complex issues and identify associated factors. The questioning mind is a huge asset in this area and countless possibilities and ideas can emerge from asking: 'What is happening?' 'When is it occurring?' 'Who is involved?' and 'Why is it transpiring?'
6. Listening – possibly the most difficult thing to do is to listen with an open and objective mind to others' points of views, ideas and suggestions. However, it is vitally important to listen and to enquire about their interpretation of patient's behaviours, motivational forces, pay-offs and recommended actions.

Taken together, these informal educative strategies, which are all grounded in practice, can contribute to the learning experience.

THE NURSE–PATIENT RELATIONSHIP

The nurse-patient relationship is a complex dynamic which is qualitatively different to other therapeutic encounters. The reasons for this include the fact that nurses are available for the patients (that is, those in inpatient care) around the clock, and that nurses tend generally to be from working-class backgrounds. They are thus perceived as being more accessible and approachable than members of the other professional groups, who are often viewed in awe. However, a downside to this in terms of violence and aggression is that this makes the nurse more vulnerable to attack and injury than are other groups. When working with violent patients, the establishment of a sound nurse–patient relationship is critical for the progression of the patient's health career and the understanding of his behaviour. The therapeutic nurse–patient relationship that is built on mutual trust and honesty will enable a careful analysis of the motivations for the aggressive action and will aid the establishment of an overall picture of the patient's behavioural repertoire. By understanding the patient, this can provide a platform for learning about his violence and can also offer indications to changes in behaviour, which may indicate prodromal signs of an impending attack.

The nurse–patient relationship should have the following themes (Brown 1986):

1. recognise individual qualities and needs
2. reassure
3. provide two-way information
4. allow the demonstration of professional expertise
5. alleviate discomfort
6. be based on quality time
7. promote autonomy
8. be vigilant to signs and symptoms.

This will form a structure for analysis of the patient's behaviour and a framework for offering interventions. Furthermore, it will contribute significantly to the learning process in relation to violence and aggression.

On a practical note, however, we should also be aware of the problems that are faced when an assault takes place. It is bad enough when we are injured by someone who is a complete stranger or whom we barely know. However, when the person who assaults us is someone with whom we have developed a therapeutic nurse–patient relationship based on respect and trust, the emotional (not to dismiss the physical) trauma is all the more powerful. We may be psychologically hurt and understandably angry. These feelings will need to be discussed and dealt with in appropriate ways, for example, through supervisory approaches mentioned above.

REVIEWS

There are a number of ways in which the violent and aggressive encounter can be evaluated in order to provide a vehicle for learning from the experience.

Critical incident analysis

Having a more structured approach to evaluating violence and aggressive incidents may help in, or contribute to, furthering our understanding of this complex behaviour. Critical incident analysis offers such a structure. It is a reflective process whereby a group of staff meet together to discuss a particular incident that occurred in clinical practice. It must, by necessity, involve those staff who were part of the incident, some who may have witnessed it, and others who act as 'sounding boards' or facilitators. There are a number of approaches to critical incident analysis, which, generally, fall along a continuum based on the extent to which the approach is student centred (Minghella & Benson 1995). However, the important point is more concerned with the focus upon the learning experience for all those involved (Burnard 1989). It is a process that was cultivated in the post Second World War era with airline pilots and is based on the personal reflection of a set of factors that are relevant to a particular incident. It was quickly adopted in other arenas in which personal feelings can confuse and confound objective analysis of a situation and affect performance in subsequent incidents. Critical incidents have been defined as: ('snapshots, vignettes, brief episodes, which epitomise a situation or an encounter which is of interest, for whatever reason' (Beattie 1987, p. 42). This lends itself neatly to the many and varied types of violent outburst and aggressive moments that can leave those involved physically and psychologically traumatised.

Criticisms of critical incident analysis

However, critical incident analysis is not without its critics. Greenwood (1993) felt that the emphasis upon verbal recollections of critical incidents were at odds with the theoretical perspectives that govern (or ought to) practice. Furthermore, she argued for more closely related practice–theory reflection that could be empirically tested. Kottkamp (1990) was also dismissive of critical incident analysis but for different reasons. This author felt that, like so many other nursing approaches: 'reflection and reflective practice may become only the latest in the casualty list of ideas with great potential that have been reduced to the level of tinkling jargon through uninformed use' (Kottkamp 1990, p. 40). However, this is more a criticism of the nursing profession than of critical incident analysis. Notwithstanding these and other sceptical points, critical incident analysis has many supporters who value it as an effective tool for reflective practice and learning from experience.

Methods

As was mentioned above, there are varyious approaches to critical incident analysis and here we present a typical method based on the work of a number of authors and our own practical experience with the technique. Qualified staff and students alike, are requested to maintain a diary or portfolio of critical incidents, which should be written up immediately after the resolution of the incident, or as soon as is practicable. The record should include:

1. Statements of fact – what happened as far as you can ascertain?
2. Statements of feeling – what did you think about the incident, what did you feel?

3. Statements of learning – what could have been done to improve the situation or prevent it occurring; what did you do that could have been done better or differently?
4. Statements of regard – what did you do well; what did others do well?

And prior to the critical incident analysis session, there should be two further statements:

5. Statements of reflection – what are your feelings now in regard to the incident?
6. Statements of sharing – what aspects of the incident do you most wish to share and why, and what aspects do you least wish to share and why?

Following the critical incident analysis meeting, the final statement should be addressed:

7. Statements of benefits – general thoughts regarding the critical incident analysis meeting, advantages and disadvantages, and how it could be improved.

The critical incident analysis structure, as outlined above, is geared towards learning from the event in order that experience is gained and possible future violent situations are avoided. This is differentiated from the critical incident stress de-briefing exercise discussed in Chapter 13 (p. 232), which was adopted as a crisis intervention to support personnel following a traumatic event.

Multidisciplinary approach

At face value, there would appear to be no particular reason why the different professions involved in the management of violence and aggression in health settings should, in fact, work together. They have very different historical developments, class structures and status divisions, not to mention particular occupational knowledge. However, a major thrust of health care provision over the previous 2 decades has been to strive for multidisciplinary working, and if the research is correct, in that violence is on the increase, and litigation also appears to be so, then multidisciplinary team working is vitally important. In reviewing violence and aggressive episodes, the multidisciplinary team must remain objective and non-judgemental, particularly in the first instance, when analysis of the facts and an exploration of values is being undertaken. Each discipline should explore its own role in contributing to the outbreak of violence and reflect upon whether any action, or inaction on its part, contributed to the present violent incident. This personal reflection lies at the heart of multidisciplinary team working and involves the process of reflexivity mentioned above. Multidisciplinary team working does not mean criticising other disciplines or attempting to scapegoat others in the event of things going wrong.

Discussions should centre on common ground for all disciplines involved and should converge on mutual objectives, shared by everyone and identified as being in the best interests of all concerned. Rather than criticise others' aims, there should be a sharing of interprofessional issues with clearly established policies of mutual collaboration. Avoid being prescriptive and advising (telling) others how they should (have) act(ed) but rather offer ways in which each profession could contribute towards the process of learning. In multidisciplinary team reviewing, there should be a collective response, but any strong dissenters should be allowed the opportunity to record their views. However, in difficult situations, 'sitting on the fence' should not be tolerated and members of the team should be requested to offer something constructive.

SWOT analysis

In practical terms, each member of the multidisciplinary team can take turns to highlight, from his perspective, the main points of the event, focusing upon the positive aspects as well as the negative ones. A 'SWOT' analysis may be considered helpful in which the strengths (S) of the incident can be highlighted and can be viewed as the positive points. Then the weaknesses (W) should be explored, which could include the lack of resources, the lack of appropriate interventions, the lack of multiprofessional input and so on. The opportunities (O) can then be outlined in which learning can take place and the aims and objectives for developments can be explored. Finally, the threats (T) are examined and could include, for example, the possibility of further violence, deterioration in therapeutic relationships, or investigation of complaints.

Contributory factor analysis

In the first three chapters of this book, we set out some of the many theories of violence and aggression and it is no coincidence as we close the final pages of the book that we are apparently coming full circle. This very much reflects not only the patterning of violence and aggression, but also our way of understanding it, coming to terms with it, and learning from the experience. In our contributing factor analysis, we may well focus on the numerous theories and ask ourselves whether these antecedents may have contributed to the violent encounter, and we hope that, perhaps, the discerning reader may be as comprehensive as this. However, on a more realistic note we offer the following contributing factor analysis framework as a practical guide to offer possible signposts towards a more complex evaluation.

Following the resolution of a violent encounter, it may well prove fruitful to attempt to identify any factors that may have contributed to the episode.

This type of analytical review is different from the others mentioned above as it attempts to focus not directly upon the violence and aggression, but on fringe, or peripheral factors, that may be causally related. For example, if a person suddenly begins to fight with another person apparently over a trivial matter, such as a seat being taken in to a particular room, at one level this may indicate a simple question of territorial claim or the structuring of domination–subordination hierarchy in the peer group. However, at other levels, it may point towards the development of an obsessive state – the simple comfort of the chair, the fact that it is the only one not in a draught, it has the best view of the television and so on. The important point is, that sometimes it is tempting to view violence and aggression as indicating a hugely complex dynamic, when a more simplistic analysis may reveal a subtle answer. Contributing factor analysis aids us in switching our attention back and forth from complex perspectives to simplistic ones.

Types of factor

In reflecting upon the contributory factors, one can divide these into a number of broad types. We can break down the analysis into the following areas.

1. Physical factors – is the person in pain, discomfort, tired, experiencing side-effects from medication, suffering from a hangover, or withdrawing from drugs?
2. Social factors – is the person lonely, needing attention, unable to form or sustain relationships, falling out with friends, or unable to socially interact? Are there sexual elements to this social dynamic, which may be causing some degree of frustration?
3. Environmental factors – is the temperature too hot, too cold, is there too much noise, is space available for the person to move to a quiet area away from the intensity of others' company, or is overcrowding an issue?
4. Contextual factors – is the person restrained by time, or been waiting a long time for a particular thing (e.g. an appointment, a letter, a drink, a discharge home!)? Is this causing acute/chronic frustration; are there special restrictions?
5. Clinical factors – is there a deterioration in mental state; is there a change in psychopathology? Are there behavioural changes?
6. Other factors – is the person under threat from peers, under pressure from family or friends, or under stress from staff?

These are merely a few of the many factors that may contribute to the deterioration to violence and the reader may well wish to add constantly to the growing number of factors in order to maintain a comprehensive range.

DEVELOPING A LEARNING CULTURE

One of the most progressive methods of learning from experience is to develop a spirit, an ethos, a culture of learning. Units, wards and hospitals that have an essence of learning, quickly develop strategies that not only keep them abreast of advances in their particular fields, but also push them to the vanguard of research and practice. They become places in which it is pleasurable to work and morale is high. They offer job opportunities and experience, and there is a feeling of worth in the establishment. In these environments, there is an abundance of activities such as workshops, seminars, conferences, research, teaching and training, with an emphasis on innovation and creativity. In short, the learning culture is the overriding feature and the counterstructures of low morale, burn-out and static practices are not tolerated. However, in moving towards this learning culture, there are a number of major obstacles that may need addressing.

In one sense, listing the factors that contribute towards a learning culture, such as reflective practice, supervision and research, is a much easier endeavour than identifying the structures that obstruct these developments. However, large groups of people who are drawn together in a common purpose tend to coalesce their behaviour around the objective that that group is set. For example, the armed forces and police have cultures based on control and discipline as part of their objectives in maintaining law and order on a national and international level. They have strong systems of discipline based on a hierarchical structuring of superior–subordinate positioning, which is emblematic of their operational practice in achieving their objectives. Similarly, psychiatric cultures have been analysed in terms of their social structures which have evolved in response to their institutional functions. Caudill et al (1952) noted how the interaction processes of a psychiatric ward operated to control patients and maintain an insular staff culture. They observed that patients were coerced into adherence to certain attitudes in four areas of life: 'toward the self, toward other patients, toward therapy and the therapist, and toward the nurses and other hospital personnel' (Caudill et al 1952, p. 317). This group focused upon the values and role systems of the culture in maintaining a ward management structure that disengaged therapy.

Goffman (1962), in his now famous essays on asylums, mapped out the sad lot of mental patients, and staff, who were locked into a totalising institution. He noted many aspects of asylum life that were perpetuated to obstruct progress and development and concluded that these asylums were little different from army camps, prison establishments, boarding schools and monasteries. Morrison (1990) exposed a strong sense of machoism in a psychiatric culture that subtly operated to foreclose on progressive developments, maintaining a self-reinforcing tradition of toughness. Furthermore, this auther highlighted culturally legitimated acts of violence by staff in the form of control and restraint of psychiatric patients, thus showing how aggression is used to manage violence. Richman & Mason (1992) outlined the development of an atypical culture in forensic psychiatry that was based in a closed, insular, macho system emanating from the institutional objectives of protecting the public whilst maintaining control of the patient's dangerous and violent behaviour.

These, then, are a few of the obstacles that must be overcome, or dismantled, in order to develop a culture of learning. Without tackling the root causes of these obstacles, a progressive spirit will not crystallise into an operational practice.

CONCLUSIONS

This chapter brings the cycle full circle, in that we conclude with the importance of learning from the experience of managing violence and aggression. Although the practices adopted in avoiding or managing such incidents are often difficult and frequently uncomfortable, we need to draw on such experiences and glean as much knowledge from them as is possible in order to prevent their occurrence in the future. We have noted how the human mind has the ability to reflect, not only on external events but also on inner feelings that exist within the mind itself. This 'bending back' of the mind upon itself affords us the opportunity of understanding violent situations in relation to previous events that are deemed similar, or typical. This growing stock of knowledge can then be applied to future encounters.

The importance of strategies to formalise learning experiences were outlined and these included the establishment of research into violence and aggression. Debates concerning the appropriateness of quantitative and qualitative research methods have been left aside, with only a passing comment to the effect that all methods were helpful in aiding our understanding. The emphasis in this chapter has been placed on the more practical-orientated method of enquiry known as action research. This approach attempts to develop practice alongside the application of research, and in one conjoint activity, bridges the theory–practice divide. Supervision techniques were also claimed to be important in the development strategy of learning, and these included clinical supervision, mentorship and leadership. Formal and informal educational approaches were then discussed and the importance of reading, writing, teaching, talking, thinking and listening have been emphasised. The trials and tribulations inherent in the formulation of therapeutic nurse–patient relationships have been examined and the significance of using this as a strategy for learning was stressed.

Reviewing of violent and aggressive encounters has been discussed in relation to critical incident analysis, multidisciplinary team working and contributing factor analysis. These approaches are crucial in learning from the experience of managing these situations. Finally, we have stressed the relevance of developing a learning culture and outlined some of the major obstacles to developing this progressive spirit. As violence and aggression lie at the soul of humankind, it will need creativity and ingenuity to overcome their aberrant manifestation.

We have attempted, in this book, to structure the contents to resemble closely a practical encounter with a violent or aggressive person. This has entailed, as would a real situation, a rapid assessment of the theory of the violence being confronted, which includes an evaluation of factors that may have contributed, or are contributing, to the situation. From this, we have undertaken observations as we approach the event, or the attacker approaches us, and we attempt de-escalation, or defusing techniques. Should the situation deteriorate, we then make decisions regarding the most appropriate intervention based on an evaluation of the current event in relation to previous ones. These interventions may be isolating the aggressive person, physically holding him, placing him in mechanical restraints, or giving him drugs to subdue him. Finally, once the situation is under control we begin our reflection upon what happened in an attempt to learn from the experience and help prevent it occurring again in the future.

Since individuals are unique, as too, are the violent and aggressive encounters that ensue from human interactions, it is clear that a definitive manual for the management of violence and aggression in all situations cannot be complete. It is therefore left to the individuals in any violent encounter to assess the most appropriate course of action, given the available resources, experience and ideology. However, what we have attempted to show in this book is that these situations are being met around the world and that they have been faced by others in the past. We have produced many references and overall principles to support the management of violence and aggression to show that in this most difficult of encounters you, and we, are not alone.

References

Abercrombie N, Hill S, Turner B S 1994 Dictionary of sociology. Penguin, London

Allon R 1971 Sex, race, social class and process-reactive schizophrenia ratings. Journal of Nervous and Mental Disease 153: 343–350

Alty A, Mason T 1994 Seclusion and mental health: a break with the past. Chapman & Hall, London

American Psychiatric Association 1989 Diagnostic and statistical manual of mental disorders, revised 3rd edn. American Psychiatric Association, Washington DC

Anderson C A 1989 Temperature and aggression: ubiquitous effects of heat on occurrence of human violence. Psychological Bulletin 106: 74–96

Angold A 1989 Seclusion. British Journal of Psychiatry 154: 437–444

Archea C, McNeely E, Martino-Saltzman D, Hennessy C, Whittington F, Myers D 1993 Restraints in long term care. Physical and Occupational Therapy in Geriatrics 11(2): 3–23

Aurelianus C 5th Century AD Madness or insanity. In: Goshen C E (ed) 1967 Documentary history of psychiatry. Vision Press, London

Averill J 1982 Anger and aggression, Springer-Verlag, Berlin

Baldwin S, Barker P 1995 Uncivil liberties: the politics of care for younger people. Journal of Mental Health 1: 41–50

Bandura A 1982 The psychology of chance encounters and life paths. American Psychologist 37: 747–755

Baradell J G 1985 Humanistic care of the patient in seclusion. Journal of Psychosocial Nursing 23(2): 9–15

Barash D A 1984 Defusing the violent patient – before he explodes. Registered Nurse March: 34–37

Beattie A 1987 Making a curriculum work. In: Allen P, Jolley M (eds) The curriculum in nursing education. Croom Helm, London

Becker E 1961 Anthropological notes on the concept of aggression. Psychiatry 25: 328–338

Belcastro P A, Gold R S, Hays L C 1983 Maslach burn-out inventory: factor structures for samples of teachers. Psychological Reports 53(2): 364–366

Berkowitz L 1986 Some varieties of human aggression: criminal violence as coercion, rule-following, impression management, and impulsive behaviour. In: Campbell A, Gibbs J J (eds) Violent transaction: the limits of personality. Blackwell, Oxford

Bernstein H A 1981 Survey of threats and assaults directed toward psychotherapists. American Journal of Psychotherapy 35: 542–549

Beskow J, Runeson B, Asgard U 1990 Psychological autopsies: methods and ethics. Suicide and Life Threatening Behavior 20: 307–323

Billig M, Condor S, Edwards D, Gane M, Middleton D, Radley A 1988 Ideological dilemmas: a social psychology of everyday thinking. Sage, London

Bjorkly S 1995 Open-area seclusion in the long-term treatment of aggressive and disruptive psychotic patients: an introduction to a ward procedure. Psychological Review 76(1): 147–157

Blackburn R 1968 Personality in relation to extreme aggression in psychiatric offenders. British Journal of Psychiatry 114: 821–828

Blackburn R 1971 Personality types among abnormal homicides. British Journal of Criminology 11: 14–31

Blackburn R 1993 The psychology of criminal conduct: theory, research and practice. John Wiley, New York

Blackburn R, Lee-Evans J M 1985 Reactions of primary and secondary psychopaths to anger evoking situations. British Journal of Clinical Psychology 24: 93–100

Bragg W D, Hoover E L, Turner E A, Nelson-Knuckles B, Weaver W L 1992 Profile of trauma due to violence in a Statewide prison population. Southern Medical Journal 85(4): 365–369
Braithwaite R 1992 Violence: understanding, intervention and prevention. Radcliffe Professional Press, Oxford
Brown L 1986 The experience of care: patient perspectives. Topics in Clinical Nursing 8(2): 56–62
Buickhuisen W, Van Der Plas-Korenhoff C, Bontekoe E H M 1988 Alcohol and violence. In: Moffitt T E, Mednick S A (eds) Biological contributions to crime causation. Martinus Nijhoff, Dordrecht
Burchard F 1988 Verlaufsstudie zur Festhaltetherapie: erste Ergebnisse bei 85 Kindern. (Process evaluation of holding therapy: preliminary results among 85 children.) Praxis der Kinderpsychologie und Kinderpsychiatrie 37(3): 89–98
Burnard P 1989 Teaching interpersonal skills: a handbook of experiential learning for health professionals. Chapman & Hall, London
Bushman B J, Cooper H M 1990 Effects of alcohol on human aggression: an integrative research review. Psychological Bulletin 107: 341–354
Buss A H 1961 The Psychology of aggression. Wiley, New York
Buunk B P, Doosje B J, Jans L G J, Hopstaken L E M 1993 Perceived reciprocity, social support, and stress at work: the role of exchange and communal orientation. Journal of Personality and Social Psychology 65(4): 801–811
Carmel H, Hunter M 1991 Psychiatrists injured by patient attack. Bulletin of the American Academy of Psychiatry and the Law 19(3): 309–316
Carney F L 1978 Inpatient treatment programs. In: Reid W H (ed) The psychopath: a comprehensive study of antisocial disorders and behaviors. Brunner/Mazel, New York
Caudill W, Redlich F C, Gilmore H R, Brody E B 1952 Social structure and interaction processes on a psychiatric ward. American Journal of Orthopsychiatry 22: 314–334
Cembrowicz S P, Shepard J P 1992 Violence in the accident and emergency department. Journal of Medicine, Science and the Law 32(2): 118–122
Chadwick R, Kroese B 1993 Do the ends justify the means? Aversive procedures in the treatment of severe challenging behaviours. In: Fleming I, Kroese B (eds) People with learning disability and severe challenging behaviour: new developments in services and therapy. Manchester University Press, Manchester
Chandley M 1995a Using verbal de-escalation techniques: celebrating good practice within forensic care. Networking, July Issue 1. SHSA, London
Chandley M 1995b Using verbal de-escalation techniques: making the vision a reality. SHSA, London
Chandley M, Mason T 1995 Nursing chronically dangerous patients. Psychiatric Care 2(1): 20–23
Cherniss C 1980 Staff burn-out: job stress in the human service organizations. Praeger, New York
Chu C-C, Ryan S J 1987 The role of seclusion in psychiatric hospital practice. Psychiatric Hospital 18(3): 121–125
Clark M, Friedman D 1992 Pulling together: building a community debriefing team. Journal of Psychosocial Nursing and Mental Health Services 30(7): 23–32
Clarke L 1995 Nursing research: science, visions and telling stories. Journal of Advanced Nursing 21: 584–593
Coid J 1982 Alcoholism and violence. Drug and Alcohol Dependence 9: 1–13
Cohen L J 1994 Psychiatric hospitalisation as an experience of trauma. Archives of Psychiatric Nursing VIII (2) (April): 78–81
COHSE (Confederation of Health Service Employees) 1977 The management of violent or potentially violent patients. COHSE, London
Coldwell J B, Naismith L 1989 Violent incidents on special care wards in a special hospital. Journal of Medicine, Science and the Law 29(2): 116–123
Colson D B, Allen J G, Coyne L, Deering D, Jehl N, Kearns W, Spohn H 1986
Profiles of difficult psychiatric hospital patients. Hospital and Community Psychiatry 37(7): 720–724
Conacher G N 1995 The use of force, chemical agents and restraint in a prison psychiatric setting. Journal of Clinical Forensic Medicine 2: 61–64
Concise Oxford dictionary of current english 1992, eighth edn. Clarendon Press, Oxford

Conolly J 1856 Treatment of the insane without mechanical restraints. Dawsons of Pall Mall, London
Cooper C 1995 Psychiatric stress debriefing: alleviating the impact of patient suicide and assault. Journal of Psychosocial Nursing 33(5): 21–25
Cortes J B, Gatti F M 1972 Delinquency and crime: a biopsychosocial approach. Seminar Press, New York
Craig C, Ray F, Hix C 1989 Seclusion and restraint: decreasing the discomfort. Journal of Psychosocial Nursing and Mental Health Services 27(7): 16–19, 31–32
Craven J L, Voore P M, Voineskos G 1987 P.r.n. medication for psychiatric inpatients. Canadian Journal of Psychiatry 32: 199–203
Crowhurst G, Carlile G, Horsfall L 1993 Gentle teaching: an introduction. Nursing Standard 7(34): 37–39
Crowner M L 1989 Current approaches to the prediction of violence. American Psychiatric Press, Washington
Crowner M L, Peric G, Tepcic F, Van-Oss E 1994a A comparison of videocameras and official incident reports in detecting inpatient assaults. Hospital and Community Psychiatry 45(11): 1144–1145
Crowner M L, Stepcic F, Peric G, Czobor P 1994b Typology of patient–patient assaults detected by videocameras. American Journal of Psychiatry 151(11): 1669–1672
Darcy P T 1985 Mental health sourcebook. Baillière Tindall, New York
Davies S 1996 Big brother. Pan Books, London
Department of Health 1997 Press release: new guidance published to combat violence in hospitals. Monday 2 June 97/21. Department of Health, London
Deschamp C 1994 Calming the demon within: chemical vs physical restraint. Journal of Emergency Medical Services 19(10): 49–53
Dewhurst K 1970 The new methods of restraint. Nursing Times 66: 749–751
Dimond B 1995 Legal aspects of nursing, 2nd edn. Prentice Hall, London
Dollard J, Miller N, Doob L, Mowrer O H, Sears R R 1939 Frustration and aggression. Yale University Press, New Haven C T
Donohue W A, Ramesh C, Borchgrevink C 1991 Crisis bargaining: tracking relational paradox in hostage negotiation. International Journal of Conflict Management 2(4): 257–274
Donohue W A, Roberto A J 1993 Relational development as negotiated order in hostage negotiation. Human Communication Research 20(2): 175–198
Dooley E 1986 Aggressive incidents in a secure hospital. Journal of Medicine, Science and the Law 26(2): 125–130
Dorsey M J, Iwata B A, Reid D H, Davis P A 1982 Protective equipment: continuous and contingent application in the treatment of self-injurious behaviour. Journal of Applied Behaviour Analysis 15: 217–230
Drummond D J, Sparr L F, Gordon G H 1989 Hospital violence reduction among high-risk patients. Journal of the American Medical Association 261(17): 2531–2534
Dubin W R 1981 Evaluating and managing the violent patient. Annals of Emergency Medicine 10(9): 481/51–484/54
Dubin W, Feld J 1989 Rapid tranquilization of the violent patient. American Journal of Emergency Medicine 7(5): 313–320
Edelwich J, Brodsky A 1980 Burn-out: stages of disillusionment in the helping profession. Human Sciences Press, New York
Edwards J G, Reid W H 1983 Violence in psychiatric facilities in Europe and the United States. In: Lion J R, Reid W H (eds) Assaults within psychiatric facilities. Grune and Stratton, Orlando FL
Evenson R C, Sletten I W, Altman H, Brown M L 1974 Disturbing behaviour: a study of incident reports. Psychiatric Quarterly 48: 266–275
Farrell G A, Gray C 1992 Aggression: a nurse's guide to therapeutic management. Scutari Press, London
Feinstein A, Dolan R 1991 Predictors of PTSD following psychlogical trauma. Psychological Medicine 21(1): 85–91
Feldman T B, Johnson P W 1995 The application of psychotherapeutic and self psychology principles to hostage negotiations. Journal of the American Academy of Psychoanalysis 23(2): 207–221

Felson R B, Steadman H J 1983 Situational factors in disputes leading to criminal violence. Criminology 21: 59–74
Ferracuti S, Palermo G B, Manfredi M 1993 Homicide between inpatients in a mental institution ward. International Journal of Offender Therapy and Comparative Criminology 37(4): 331–337
Feschbach S 1970 Aggression. In: Mussen P H (ed) Carmichael's manual of child psychology, vol II. Wiley, New York
Feshbach S, Price J 1984 The development of cognitive competencies and the control of aggression. Aggressive Behaviour 10: 185–200
Fishel A, Ferreiro B, Rynerson B, Nickell M, Jackson B, Hannan B 1994 As-needed psychotropic medications: prevalence, indications, and results. Journal of Psychosocial Nursing 32(8): 27–32
Fisher W A 1994 Restraint and seclusion: a review of the literature. American Journal of Psychiatry 151(11): 1584–1591
Fisher W H, Geller J L, White C L, Altaffer F 1995 Serving the seriously mentally ill in the 'least restrictive alternative': issues for a federal court consent decree. Administration and Policy in Mental Health 22(4): 423–436
Folkman S, Lazarus R (1988) Coping as a mediator of emotion. Journal of Personality and Social Psychology 54: 466–475
Fottrell E 1980 A study of violent behaviour among patients in psychiatric hospitals. British Journal of Psychiatry 136: 216–221
Foucault M 1967 Madness and civilization: a history of insanity in the age of reason. Tavistock, London
Foucault M 1978 About the concept of the 'dangerous individual' in 19th century legal psychiatry. International Journal of Law and Psychiatry 1: 1–18
Freud S 1920 Beyond the pleasure principle. In: Strachey J (ed) The complete psychological works of Sigmund Freud, vol 18. Hogarth Press, London
Freudenberger H J, Richelson G 1980 Burn-out: the high cost of high achievement. Anchor Press, New York
Gair D S 1980 Limit-setting and seclusion in the psychiatric hospital. Psychiatric Opinion 17: 15–19
Garai J E 1970 Sex differences in mental health nursing. Genetic Psychological Monograms 81: 123–142
Gates B, Wray J, Newell R 1996 Focus on learning disability nursing: challenging behaviour in children with learning disabilities. British Journal of Nursing 5(19): 1189–1194
Geen R G, O'Neil E C 1976 Perspectives on aggression. Academic Press, New York
Gentilin J 1987 Room restriction: a therapeutic prescription. Journal of Psychosocial Nursing 25(7): 12–16
Gerbi L 1994 Spousal violence: understanding and intervention techniques. Journal of Family Psychotherapy 5(4): 19–31
Gerlock A, Solomons H C 1983 Factors associated with the seclusion of psychiatric patients. Perspectives in Psychiatric Care 21(2): 47–53
Gibson D 1994 Time for clients: temporal aspects of community psychiatric nursing. Journal of Advanced Nursing 20: 110–116
Gilmartin K M, Gibson R J 1985 Hostage negotiation: the bio-behavioral dimension. The Police Chief June: 46–48
Goffman E 1962 Asylums: essays on the social situation of mental patients and other inmates. Penguin, London
Goldstein A P, Glick B 1987 Behaviour therapy. In: Corsins R (ed) Current psychotherapies. FE Peacock, Illinois
Goldstein P J 1989 Drugs and violent crime. In: Weiner N A, Wolfgang M E (eds) Pathways to criminal violence. Sage, Newbury Park CA.
Gostin L 1986 A practical guide to mental health law. MIND, London
Grayboys T B 1986 Burn-out in the care and management of survivors of out-of-hospital cardiac arrest. American Heart Journal 112(2): 428–430
Graves R 1986 Mythology. Guild Publishing, London
Greaves A 1994 Organisational approaches to the prevention and management of violence. In: Wykes T (ed) Violence and health care professionals. Chapman & Hall, London

Greenberg M S, Westcott D R 1983 Indebtedness as a mediator or reactions to aid. In: Fisher J D, Nadler A, DePaulo B M (eds) New directions in helping behavior. Academic Press, San Diego CA

Greenwood J 1993 Reflective practice: a critique of the work of Argyris and Schon. Journal of Advanced Nursing 18: 1183–1187

Gudjonsson G, Drinkwater J 1986 Intervention techniques for violent behaviour. Issues in Criminal and Legal Psychiatry 9: 37–47

Gutheil T 1978 Observations on the theoretical bases for seclusion of the psychiatric in-patient. American Journal of Psychiatry 135: 325–328

Gutheil T, Daly M 1980 Clinical considerations in seclusion room design. Hospital and Community Psychiatry 31(4): 268–270

Gutheil T, Appelbaum P, Wexler D 1983 The inappropriateness of 'least restrictive alternative' analysis for involuntary procedures with the institutionalized mentally ill. Journal of Psychiatry and Law 7: 10–15

Haffke E A, Reid W H 1983 Violence against mental health personnel in Nebraska. In: Lion J, Reid W H (eds) Assaults within psychiatric facilities. Grune & Stratton, New York

Hafner H, Boker W 1982 Crimes of violence by mentally abnormal offenders. Cambridge University Press, Cambridge

Haller R M, DeLuty R H 1988 Assaults on staff by psychiatric inpatients: a critical review. British Journal of Psychiatry 152: 174–179

Hanson R H, Balk J A 1992 A replication study of staff injuries in a State Hospital. Hospital and Community Psychiatry 43(8): 836–837

Harris G T, Rice M E, Quinsey V L 1993 Violent recidivism of mentally disordered offenders: the development of a statistical prediction instrument. Criminal Behaviour and Mental Health 25(4): 288–294

Harris J 1996 Physical restraint procedures for managing challenging behaviours presented by mentally retarded adults and children. Research in Developmental Disabilities 17(2): 99–134

Hatti S, Dubin W R 1982 A study of the circumstances surrounding patient assaults on psychiatrists. Hospital and Community Psychiatry 33: 660–661

Hay D, Cromwell R 1980 Reducing the use of full-leather restraints on an acute adult inpatient ward. Hospital and Community Psychiatry 31: 198–200

Her Majesty's Stationery Office 1974 Health and Safety at Work Act. HMSO, London

Her Majesty's Stationery Office 1983 The Mental Health Act. HMSO, London

Her Majesty's Stationery Office 1990 Mental Act Commission: code of practice. HMSO, London

Her Majesty's Stationery Office 1992 The management of Health and Safety at Work Regulations Act. HMSO, London

Her Majesty's Stationery Office 1993. Code of practice. HMSO, London

Herbel K 1990 Management of agitated head-injured patients: a survey of current techniques. Rehabilitation Nursing 15(2): 66–69

Hickerson J, Garrison M 1991 Quiet room utilization patterns. Residential Treatment for Children and Youth 9(1): 39–49

Higgs J, Titchen A 1995 The nature, generation and verification of knowledge. Physiotherapy 81(9): 521–530

Hill J, Spreat S 1987 Staff injury rates associated with the implementation of contingent restraint. Mental Retardation 25(3): 141–145

Hodgkinson P 1985 The use of seclusion. Journal of Medicine, Science and the Law 25(3): 215–222

Hodgkinson P E, McIvor L, Phillips M 1985 Patient assaults on staff in a psychiatric hospital: a two-year retrospective study. Journal of Medicine, Science and the Law 25(4): 288–294

Horowitz M 1986 Stress response syndromes, 2nd edn. Jason Aronson, New York

Huesmann L R, Eron L D, Yarmel P W 1987 Intellectual functioning and aggression. Journal of Personality and Social Psychology 52: 232–240

Hunter M, Carmel H 1992 The cost of staff injuries from inpatient violence. Hospital and Community Psychiatry 43(6): 586–588

Ionno J A 1983 A prospective study of assaultive behaviour in female psychiatric inpatients. In: Lion J R, Reid W H (eds) Assaults within psychiatric facilities, Grune & Stratton, Orlando FL

Jambunathen J, Bellaire K 1996 Evaluating staff of crisis prevention/intervention techniques: a pilot study. Issues in Mental Health Nursing 17(6): 541–558
Joshi P T, Capozzoli J A, Coyle J T 1988 Use of a quiet room on an inpatient unit. American Academy of Child and Adolescent Psychiatry 27: 642–644
Judge W Q, Millar A 1991 Antecedents and outcomes of decision speed in different environmental contexts. Academy of Management Journal 34(2): 449–463
Justic M 1993 Restraint/seclusion: an approach to documentation and assessment. Nursing Quality Connect 2(4): 6–7
Kemmis S, McTaggart R 1982 The action research planner, 2nd edn. Deakin University Press, Victoria
Kendrick D, Wilber G 1986 Seclusion: organising safe and effective care. Journal of Psychosocial Nursing 24(11): 26–28
Kingdon D G, Bakewell E W 1988 Aggressive behaviour: evaluation of a non-seclusion policy of a district psychiatric service. British Journal of Psychiatry 153: 631–634
Kinkle S L 1993 Violence in the ED: how to stop it before it starts. American Journal of Nursing July (7): 22–24
Kinsella C, Chaloner C, Brosnan C 1993 An alternative to seclusion? Nursing Times 89(18): 62–64
Kinzel A F 1979 Body-buffer zone in violent prisoners. American Journal of Psychiatry 127: 59–64
Kirchner E, Kennedy R, Draguns J 1979 Assertion and aggression in adult offenders. Behavior Therapy 10: 452–471
Kirk A 1989 The prediction of violent behaviour during short-term civil commitment. Bulletin of American Academy of Psychiatry and Law 17(4): 345–353
Kolvin I, Miller F J W, Fleeting M, Kolvin P A 1988 Social and parenting factors affecting criminal offence rates: findings from the Newcastle Thousand Family Study (1947–1980) British Journal of Psychiatry 152: 80–90
Kottkamp R 1990 Means for facilitating reflection. Education and Urban Society 22(2): 182–203
Kraus S, Wilkenfeld J 1993 A strategic negotiations model with applications to an international crisis. IEEE Transactions on Systems, Man and Cybernetics 23(1): 313–323
Kutash S B 1978 Psychoanalytic theories of aggression. In: Kutash I L, Kutash S B, Schlesinger L B (eds) Violence: perspectives on murder and aggression. Jossey-Bass, San Francisco
LaGaipa J J 1977 Interpersonal attraction and social exchange. In: Duck S (ed) Theory and practice in interpersonal attraction. Academic Press, San Diego CA
Lambert E W, Cartor R, Walker L 1985 Reliability of behavioural versus medical models: rare events and danger. Issues in Mental Health Nursing 9: 31–44
Landau T J, MacLeish R 1988 When does time-out become seclusion, and what must be done when this line is crossed? Residential Treatment for Children and Youth 6(2): 33–38
Lanza M L 1983 The reactions of nursing staff to physical assault by a patient. Hospital and Community Psychiatry 34(1): 44–47
Lanza M L, Milner J 1989 The dollar cost of patient assault. Hospital and Community Psychiatry 40: 1227–1229
Lanza M L, Kayne H, Hicks C, Milner J 1991 Nursing staff characteristics related to patient assault. Issues in Mental Health Nursing 12(3): 253–265
Larkin E, Murtagh S, Jones S 1988 A preliminary study of violent incidents in a special hospital (Rampton). British Journal of Psychiatry 153: 226–231
Lazarus R S 1991 Cognition and motivation in emotion. American Psychologist 46: 352–367
Lazarus R S, Folkman S 1984 Stress, Appraisal and Coping. Springer, Berlin
Leadbetter D, Paterson B 1995 De-escalating aggression. In: Kidd B, Stark C (eds) Management of violence and aggression in health care. Royal College of Psychiatry, London
Leng R 1987 Structure and action in militarized disputes. In: Herman C, Kegley C, Rosenau J (eds) New directions in the study of foreign policy. Allen and Unwin, Winchester MA
Levi M 1994 Violent crime. In: Maguire M, Morgan R, Reiner R (eds) The Oxford handbook of criminology. Clarendon Press, Oxford
Lewin K 1946 Action research and minority problems. Journal of Social Issues 2: 34–46
Lidberg L, Levander S E, Schalling D, Lidberg Y 1976 Excretion of adrenaline and

noradrenaline as related to real life stress and psychopathy. Reports from the Laboratory for Clinical Stress Research, Stockhom, no. 50
Lieber A L, Sherin C R 1972 Homicides and the lunar cycle: toward a theory of lunal influences on human emotional disturbance. American Journal of Psychiatry 129: 69–74
Lion J R, Pasternak S A 1973 Countertransference in violent patients. American Journal of Psychiatry 130: 207–209
Lion J R, Snyder W, Merrill G L 1981 Underreporting of assaults on staff in a state hospital. Hospital and Community Psychiatry 32: 497–498
Littlewood R, Lipsedge M 1989 Aliens and alienists: ethnic minorities and psychiatry. Unwin Hyman, London
Lorenz K 1966 On aggression. Methuen, London
Lynch T G, Fuller R 1994 Playing with fire: negotiating with the homicidal/suicidal patient. Topics in Emergency Medicine 16(3): 44–52
MacCulloch M J, Bailey J 1991 Issues in the provision and evaluation of forensic services. Journal of Forensic Psychiatry 2: 247–265
McDonell A A, Sturmey P, Dearden B 1993 The acceptability of physical restraint procedures for people with a learning difficulty. Behavioural and Cognitive Psychotherapy 21: 255–264
McLaren S, Browne F, Taylor P 1990 A study of psychotropic medication given 'as required' in a regional secure unit. British Journal of Psychiatry 156: 732–735
Madden D J, Lion J, Penna M W 1976 Assaults on psychiatrists by patients. American Journal of Psychiatry 133: 422–425
Maier G J, Van Rybroek G J 1990 Offensive images: managing aggression isn't pretty. Hospital and Community Psychiatry 41(4): 357
Maier G J, Stava L J, Morrow B R, Van Rybroek G J, Bauman K G 1987 A model for understanding and managing cycles of aggression among psychiatric inpatients. Hospital and Community Psychiatry 38(5): 520–524
Maier G J, Van Rybroek G J, Doren D, Musholt E A, Miller R D 1988 A comprehensive model for understanding and managing aggressive inpatients. American Journal of Continuing Education in Nursing section C: 1–18
Maksymchuk A F 1982 Strategies for hostage-taking incidents. Police Chief April: 58–65
Marra H A, Konzelman G E, Giles P G (1987) A clinical strategy to the assessment of dangerousness. International Journal of Offender Therapy and Comparative Criminology 31: 291–299
Marsh I 1994 Sociology in focus: crime. Longman, London
Maslach C 1982 Understanding burn-out: definitional issues in analyzing a complex phenomenon. In: Paine W S (ed) Job stress and burn-out: research, theory and intervention perspectives. Sage, London
Maslach C, Jackson S E 1978 Lawyer burn-out. Barrister 8: 52–58
Mason A A, DeWolfe A S 1974 Usage of psychotropic drugs in a mental hospital: as needed (p.r.n.) antipsychotic medications. Current Therapeutic Research 16: 853–860
Mason T 1993a Seclusion theory reviewed: a benevolent or malevolent intervention. Journal of Medicine, Science and the Law 33(2): 95–102
Mason T 1993b Seclusion: international comparisons. Journal of Medicine, Science and the Law 34(1): 54–60
Mason T 1993c Seclusion as a cultural practice in a special hospital. Educational Action Research 1(3): 411–423
Mason T 1993d Special hospital seclusion and its clinical variations. Journal of Clinical Nursing 2: 95–102
Mason T 1994 Legal aspects and policy issues. In: Alty A, Mason T (eds) Seclusion and mental health: a break with the past. Chapman & Hall, London
Mason T 1995 Seclusion in the special hospitals: a descriptive and analytical study. SHSA, London
Mason T 1996a Scatolia: psychosis to protest. Journal of Psychiatric and Mental Health Nursing 3: 303–311
Mason T 1996b Seclusion and learning difficulties: research and deductions. British Journal of Developmental Disabilities 62(2): 149–159
Mason T, Hennighan M, Chandley M, Johnson D 1996 Decompression of long-term seclusion. Psychiatric Care 3(6): 217–225

Mason T 1997 Seclusion and the lunar cycles. Journal of Psychosocial Nursing 35(6): 14–18
Mason T, Chandley M 1995 The chronically assaultive patient: benchmarking best practices. Psychiatric Care 2(5): 180–183
Mattson J L, Keyes J 1988 Contingent reinforcement and contingent restraint to treat severe aggression and self-injury in mentally retarded and autistic adults. Journal of the Multihandicapped Person 1(2): 141–153
Mayhew P, Elliott D, Dowds L 1989 The 1988 British crime survey. HMSO, London
Mazaleski J L, Iwata B A, Rodgers T A, Vollmer T R, Zarcone J R 1994 Protective equipment as treatment for stereotypic hand mouthing: sensory extinction or punishment effects? Journal of Applied Behaviour Analysis 27(2): 345–355
Mead G H 1934 Mind, self and society. University of Chicago Press, Chicago
Megargee E I 1966 Undercontrolled and overcontrolled personality types in extreme antisocial aggression. Psychological Monographs 80: no. 611
Melchior M E W, Philipsen H, Huyer Abu-Saad H, Halfens R J G, Van de Berg A, Gassman P 1996 The effectiveness of primary nursing on burnout among psychiatric nurses in long-stay settings. Journal of Advanced Nursing 24: 694–702
Mendoza R, Djenderedjian A H, Adams J 1987 Midazolan in acute psychotic patients with hyperarousal. Journal of Clinical Psychiatry 48: 291–292
Merton R K 1939 Social structure and anomie. American Sociological Review 3: 672–682
Miles S H 1993 Restraints and sudden death. Journal of the Gerontological Society 41(9): 1013
Miller D E 1986 The management of misbehaviour by seclusion. Residential Treatment for Children and Youth 4(1): 63–73
Miller D, Walker M C, Friedman D 1989 Use of a holding technique to control the violent behavior of seriously disturbed adolescents. Hospital and Community Psychiatry 40(5): 520–524
Mills H 1994 Private sector to supervise tagging of criminals. *The Independent* 22 September, London
Minghella E, Benson A 1995 Developing reflective practice in mental health nursing through critical incident analysis. Journal of Advanced Nursing 21(2): 205–213
Molasiotis A 1995 Use of physical restraints 2: alternatives. British Journal of Nursing 4(4): 201–220
Monahan J 1984 The prediction of violent behaviour: toward a second generation of theory and policy. American Journal of Psychiatry 141: 10–15
Monroe C M, Van Rybroek G, Maier G 1988 Decompressing agressive inpatients: breaking the aggression cycle to enhance positive outcome. Behavioural Sciences and the Law 6(4): 543–557
Monroe R 1978 Brain dysfunction in aggressive criminals. Heath, Lexington
Moran T, Mason T 1996 Revisiting the nursing management of the psychopath. Journal of Psychiatric and Mental Health Nursing 3(3): 189–194
Morrison E F 1990 The tradition of toughness: a study of nonprofessional nursing care in psychiatric settings. Image: Journal of Nursing Scholarship 22(1): 32–38
Morrison P 1991 The use of environmental seclusion monitored. Nursing Times 87(37): 54
Moyer K 1981 Biological substrates of aggression: implications for control. In: Brain P F, Benton D (eds) The biology of aggression. Sijthoff and Noordhoff, Alphen aan der Rijn
Mueller C W 1983 Environmental stressors and agressive behavior. In: Geen R G, Donnerstein E I (eds) Aggression: theoretical and empirical reviews, vol 2. Academic Press, New York
Musisi S M, Wasylenki D A, Rapp M S 1989 A psychiatric intensive care unit in a psychiatric hospital. Canadian Journal of Psychiatry 34(3): 200–204
Musker M 1992 Making contact. Nursing Times 88(47): 31–33
Nagy S 1985 Burn-out and selected variables as components of occupational stress. Psychological Reports 56(1): 195–200
Neufeld A, Fantuzzo J W 1984 Contingent application of a protective device to treat the severe self-biting behaviour of a disturbed autistic child. Journal of Behaviour Therapy and Experimental Psychiatry 15: 79–83
Noble P, Rogers S 1989 Violence by psychiatric in-patients. British Journal of Psychiatry 155: 384–390
Novaco R W 1975 Anger control. Lexington, Toronto

Novaco R W 1978 Anger and coping with stress. In: Foreyt J P, Rathjen D P (eds) Cognitive behaviour therapy. Plenum, New York
Nurco D N, Ball J C, Shaffer J W, Hanlon E 1985 The criminality of narcotic addicts. Journal of Nervous and Mental Disease 173: 94–102
Okin R L 1985 Variation among state hospitals in use of seclusion. Hospital and Community Psychiatry 36: 648–652
O'Neil E, Brunault M, Marquis J, Carifio M 1979 Anger and the body buffer zone. Journal of Social Psychology 108: 135–136
Outlaw F, Lowery B 1994 An attributional study of seclusion and restraint of psychiatric patients. Archives of Psychiatric Nursing 8(2): 69–77
Oxford English Dictionary 1990 Oxford University Press, Oxford
Palmistierna T, Wistedt B 1995 Changes in the pattern of aggressive behaviour among inpatients with changed ward organisation. Acta Psychiatrica Scandinavica 91: 32–35
Paterson B, Leadbetter D 1995 Dealing with a hostage situation. Nursing Times 91(3): 28–29
Pearson G 1983 Hooliganism: a history of respectable fears. Macmillan, London
Pearson M, Wilmot E, Padi M 1986 A study of violent behaviour among in-patients in a psychiatric hospital. British Journal of Psychiatry 149: 232–235
Pernanen K 1991 Alcohol in human violence. Guilford, New York
Phillips D, Rudestam K E 1995 Effect of nonviolent self-defense training on male psychiatric members' aggression and fear. Psychiatric Services 46(2): 164–168
Pines A, Aronson E 1981 Burn-out: from tedium to personal growth. Free Press, New York
Piotrowski K W 1979 Physical restraints or rapid neuroleptization? Journal of the Florida Medical Association 66: 924–926
Pitt B 1987 Exercising restraints. International Journal of Gerontological Psychiatry 2(4): 207–210
Plous S 1993 The psychology of judgement and decision making. McGraw-Hill, New York
Powell M K 1991 Hostage-situation policy statement for the emergency department. Journal of Emergency Nursing 17(5): 313–315
Poyner B, Warne C 1986 Violence to staff: a basis for assessment and prevention. HMSO, London
Randell B, Walsh E 1994 The verdict is in: seclusion is out: Journal of Child and Adolescent Nursing 7(4): 3–4
Rapoport R N 1970 Three dilemmas in action research. Human Relations 23(6): 499–513
Rasmussen K, Levander S 1996 Individual rather than situational characteristics predict violence in a maximum security hospital. Journal of Interpersonal Violence 11: 12–19
Ratey J J, Leveroni C, Kilmer D, Gutheil C, Swartz B 1993 The effects of clozapine on severely aggressive psychiatric inpatients in a state hospital. Journal of Clinical Psychiatry 54(6): 219–223
Ray N, Rappaport M 1995 Use of restraints and seclusion in psychiatric settings in New York State. Psychiatric Services 56(10): 1032–1037
Reid W H, Kang J S 1986 Serious assaults by out-patients or former patients. American Journal of Psychotherapy 40: 594–600
Resnick M, Burton B T 1984 Droperidol vs haloperidol in the initial management of acutely agitated patients. Journal of Clinical Psychiatry 45: 298–299
Rice M E, Harris G T, Varney G W, Quinsey V L 1989 Violence in institutions: understanding, prevention and control. Hogrefe & Huber, Toronto
Richman J 1998 Ceremonial and moral order of a ward for psychopaths. In: Mason T, Mercer D (eds) Critical perspectives in forensic care. Macmillan, London
Richman J, Mason T 1992 Quo vadis the special hospitals? In: Scott S, Williams G, Platt S, Thomas H (eds) Private risks and public dangers. Averbury, Aldershot
Rittman M 1993 Social organisation of length of stay of psychiatric patients. Journal of Psychosocial Nursing 31: 21–27
Robinson B E, Sucholeiki R, Schocken D D 1993 Sudden death and resisted mechanical restraint: a case report. Journal of the American Gerontological Society 41: 424–425
Rolfe G 1990 The role of clinical approach. Nurse Education Today 10: 193–197
Roth J A 1963 Timetables: structuring the passage of time in hospital treatment and other careers. Bobbs-Merrill, New York
Rotten J, Frey J 1985 Air pollution, weather, and violent crimes: concomitant time-series analysis of archival data. Journal of Personality and Social Psychology 49: 1207–1220
Royal College of Nursing 1972 Care of the violent patient. RCN, London

Royal College of Nursing 1994 Issues in nursing and health: the privacy of clients: electronic tagging and closed circuit television March RCN, London
Ruben I, Wolkon G, Yamamoto J 1980 Physical attacks on psychiatric residents by patients. Journal of Nervous and Mental Disease 168: 243–245
Saks E 1986 The use of mechanical restraints in psychiatric hospitals. Yale Law Journal 95(8): 1836–1856
Salvatore N G 1993 Restraints: a sampling of current practice. Journal of Emergency Nursing 19: 417–421
Samter J, Fitzgerald M L, Braudaway C A, Leeks D, Padgett M B, Swartz A L, Gary-Stephens M, Dellinger N F 1993 Debriefing: from military origin to therapeutic application. Journal of Psychosocial Nursing and Mental Health Services 31(2): 23–27
Schalling D, Asberg M, Adman G, Oreland L 1987 Markers for vulnerability to psychopathology: temperament traits associated with platelet MAO activity. Acta Psychiatrica Scandinavica 76: 172–182
Schneidman E S 1969 Suicide, lethality and the psychological autopsy. International Psychiatry Clinics 6: 255–259
Schutz A 1970 On phenomenology and social relations. University of Chicago Press, Chicago
Schwab P J, Lahmeyer C B 1979 The use of seclusion on a general hospital psychiatric unit. Journal of Clinical Psychiatry 40: 228–231
Sclafani M 1986 Violence and behaviour control. Journal of Psychosocial Nursing 24(11): 8–13
Selby M J 1984 Assessment of violence potential using measures of anger, hostility, and social desirability. Journal of Personality Assessment 48: 531–544
Severinsson E I 1994 The concept of supervision in psychiatric care-compared with mentorship and leadership: a review of the literature. Journal of Nursing Management 2: 271–278
Shader R I, Jackson A H, Hartmatz J S 1977 Patterns of violent behaviour among schizophrenic inpatients. Disorders of the Nervous System 38: 13–16
Sheline Y, Nelson T 1993 Patient choice: deciding between psychotropic medication and physical restraints in an emergency. Bulletin of the American Academy of Psychiatry and the Law 21(3): 321–329
Singh N N, Dawson M J, Manning P J 1981 The effect of physical restraint on self-injurious behaviour. Journal of Mental Deficiency Research 25: 207–216
Snyder G H, Diesling P 1977 Conflict among nations: bargaining, decision making and system structure in international crises. Princeton University Press, Princeton NJ
Special Hospitals Service Authority 1993 The use of seclusion and the alternative management of disturbed behaviour within the special hospitals. The Special Hospitals Service Authority, London
Starrin B, Larsson G, Styrborn S 1990 A review and critique of psychological approaches to the burn-out phenomenon. Scandinavian Journal of Caring Sciences 4(2): 83–91
Stermac L E 1986 Anger control treatment for forensic patients. Journal of Interpersonal Violence 1: 446–457
Stevenson S 1991 Heading off violence with verbal de-escalation. Journal of Psychosocial Nursing 29(9): 6–10
Stirling C, McHugh A 1997 Natural therapeutic holding: a non-aversive alternative to the use of control and restraint in the management of violence for people with learning disabilities. Journal of Advanced Nursing 26(2): 304–311
Stolley J 1995 Freeing your patients from restraints. American Journal of Nursing 27: 31
Stolley J, King J, Clarke M, Joers A M, Hague D, Allen D 1993 Developing a restraint use policy for acute care. Journal of Nursing Administration 23(12): 49–54
Strawser D 1994 Restraint and seclusion record. Journal of Emergency Nursing 20(5): 404
Tanke E D, Yesavage J A 1985 Characteristics of assaultive patients who do and do not provide visible cues of potential violence. American Journal of Psychiatry 141: 1232–1235
Tardiff K 1981 Assaults in hospital and placement in the community. Bulletin of the American Academy of Psychiatry and the Law 93: 33–39
Tardiff K 1989 Assessment and management of violent patients. American Psychiatric Press, London
Tardiff K 1992 Mentally abnormal offenders: evaluation and management of violence. Psychiatric Clinics of North America 15(3): 553–567

Tardiff K, Sweillam W 1982 Assaultive behaviour among chronic psychiatric inpatients. American Journal of Psychiatry 139: 212–215
Taylor A D, Sinclair A, Wall E M 1987 Sources of stress in postgraduate medical training. Journal of Medical Education 62(5): 425–428
Taylor P 1982 Schizophrenia and violence. In: Gunn J, Farrington D P (eds) Abnormal offenders, delinquency, and the criminal justice system. John Wiley, New York
Taylor P 1985 Motives for offending among violent and psychotic men. British Journal of Psychiatry 147: 491–498
Tedeschi J T 1983 Social influence theory and aggression. In: Geen R G, Donnerstein E I (eds) Aggression: theoretical and empirical reviews, vol 1. Academic Press, New York
Toch H 1969 Violent men. Penguin, Harmondsworth
Topf M 1988 Verbal interpersonal responsiveness. Journal of Psychosocial Nursing 26(7): 9–16
Tronick E Z 1995 Touch in mother-infant interaction. In: Tiffany M (ed) Touch in early development. Lawrence Erlbaum Associates. New Jersey
Turner J T 1984 Role of the ED nurse in health care-based hostage incidents. Journal of Emergency Nursing 10(4): 190–193
Turner P M, Turner T J 1991 Validation of the crisis triage rating scale for psychiatric emergencies. Canadian Journal of Psychiatry 36: 651–654
UKCC 1992 Code of professional conduct. UKCC, London
UKCC 1996 Guidelines for professional practice. UKCC, London
Van Rybroek G J, Kuhlman T L, Maier G J, Kaye M S 1987 Preventive aggression devices (PADs): ambulatory restraints as an alternative to seclusion. Journal of Clinical Psychiatry 48(10): 401–405
Van Rybroek G J, Maier G J, McCormick D J, Pollack D 1988 Today–tomorrow behavioural programming: realistic reinforcement for repetitively aggressive inpatients. American Journal of Continuing Education in Nursing 4:1–12
Veninga R L, Spradley J P 1981 The work stress connection. Little Brown, Boston
Virkunnen M 1988 Cerebrospinal fluid: monoamine metabolites among habitually violent and impulsive offenders. In: Moffitt T E, Mednick S A (eds) Biological contributions to crime causation. Martinus Nijhoff, Dordrecht
Vorster, de W 1990 'Holding' as a therapeutic manoeuvre in family therapy. Journal of Family Therapy 12(2): 189–194
Walster E, Walster G W, Berscheid E 1978 Equity: theory and research. Allyn & Bacon, Boston
Warneke L 1986 A psychiatric intensive care unit in a general hospital setting. Canadian Journal of Psychiatry 31(9): 834–837
Warren N, Jahoda A 1973 Attitudes. Penguin, Harmondsworth
Weick M D 1992 Physical restraints: an FDA update. American Journal of Nursing 92: 74–80
Weinberg M H, Buford C C, Bird I F, Rotov M 1970 The clinical use of chemical mace. Journal of the Medical Society of New Jersey 67: 103
West D J 1982 Delinquency: its roots, careers and prospects. Harvard University Press, Cambridge MA
Westermeyer J, Kroll J 1978 Violence and mental illness in a peasant society: characteristics of violent behaviours and 'folk' use of restraints. British Journal of Psychiatry 133: 529–541
Whittington R, Mason T 1995 A new look at seclusion: stress, coping and the perception of threat. Journal of Forensic Psychiatry 6(2): 285–304
Whittington R, Patterson P 1995 Verbal and non-verbal behaviour immediately prior to aggression by mentally disordered people: enhancing the assessment of risk. Journal of Psychiatric and Mental Health Nursing 3: 47–54
Whittington R, Wykes T 1992 Staff strain and social support in a psychiatric hospital following assault by a patient. Journal of Advanced Nursing 17: 480–486
Whittington R, Wykes T 1994a An observational study of associations between nurse behaviour and violence in psychiatric hospitals. Journal of Psychiatric and Mental Health Nursing 1: 85–92
Whittington R, Wykes T 1994b The prediction of violence in a health care setting. In: Wykes T (ed) Violence and health care professionals. Chapman & Hall, London
Whittington R, Shuttleworth S, Hill L 1996 Violence to staff in a general hospital setting. Journal of Advanced Nursing 24: 326–333
Wicker A W 1969 Attitudes v action: the relationship of verbal and overt responses to attitude objects. Journal of Social Issues 25: 41–78

Widom C S, Ames A 1988 Biology and female crime. In: Moffitt T E, Mednick S A (eds) Biological contributions to crime causation. Martinus Nijhoff, Dordrecht

Williams L M, Morton G A, Patrick C H 1990 The emory cubicle bed: an alternative to restraints for agitated traumatically brain injured clients. Rehabilitation Nursing 15(1): 30–33

Wilson E O 1978 On human nature. Harvard University Press, Cambridge MA

Winter R 1989 Learning from experience. Falmer Press, London

Wolfgang M E 1957 Victim-precipitated criminal homicide. Journal of Criminal Law, Criminology and Police Science 48: 1–11

Wolfgang M E, Ferracutti F 1967 The subculture of violence. Tavistock, London

Wong S E, Floyd J, Innocent A J, Woolsey J E 1991 Applying a DRO and compliance training to reduce aggressive and self injurious behaviour in an autistic man: a case report. Journal of Behaviour Therapy and Experimental Psychiatry 22(4): 299–304

Wykes T 1994 (ed) Violence and health care professionals. Chapman & Hall, London

Wykes T, Whittington R 1994 Reactions to assault. In: Wykes T (ed) Violence and health care professionals. Chapman & Hall, London

Zerubavel E 1987 The language of time: toward a semiotics of temporality. The Sociological Quarterly 28(3): 343–356

Zillman D 1979 Hostility and aggression. Erlbaum, Hillsdale, NJ

Zimbardo P G 1970 The human choice: individuation, reason, and order versus deindivuation, impulse and chaos. In: Arnold W J, Levine D (eds), Nebraska symposium on motivation. University of Nebraska Press, Lincoln

Index

Numbers in bold refer to illustrations and tables